Avishay Gershony M.D.

Healing Illness and Karma
An Anthroposophic Approach

According to Rudolf Steiner's Teachings

Astrolog Publishing House Ltd

Cover Design: Na'ama Yaffe

© Astrolog Publishing House Ltd. 2004

P. O. Box 1123, Hod Hasharon 45111, Israel
Tel: 972-9-7412044
Fax: 972-9-7442714

ISBN 965-494-192-9

Published by
Astrolog Publishing House 2004

To Orna,
who gave everything

Contents

Preface

How is illness linked to human life?
When does healing occur?
What is destiny or karma?

The answers offered by this book are taken from Anthroposophy, a spiritual world view whose foundations were laid by Rudolf Steiner a century ago. Although it was devised a long time ago, it is indispensable for anyone who wants to have a greater understanding of himself and his surroundings.

When a person finds out that he has an illness, he is bound to ask himself difficult questions – existential questions. The illness spurs him on to discover qualities within his soul that he did not know he possessed. It opens up a new outlook on the world for him. Every day, in my capacity as a physician, I meet people who are afflicted with a serious disease or disability. The precious soul and spiritual gifts these people have given me have made it possible to transform the thoughts and images taken from books into a living reality.

This book is meant for anyone who asks himself existential questions – first and foremost for people who themselves have a serious illness, or someone close to them has a serious illness. People who treat others – therapists, nurses and physicians – might also find this book inspiring and helpful.

The book may be difficult to read, especially for someone who is encountering the world of anthroposophic terms for the first time. In order to get the most out of the book, more concentration and attention are required than for normal, easy reading.

I would like to express my deepest thanks to Noemi Leck for her comments, which made the book more solid and a bit more readable; to Marion Duman for her good will and tremendous help; to Sandy, my wife, who with a lot of patience helped me to reduce the inaccuracies and ambiguities in the text; and to my beloved Talia and Daniel.

Introduction

The perception of illness today and in the past

The moment in which the realization of being ill permeates a person's consciousness – the realization that an illness is residing in his body and is liable to limit him in various ways and even threaten his life – is possibly the hardest moment he has ever experienced in his life. The contemporary person, who has been raised in the materialistic culture of the West, lives in an environment that attempts to distance illness from the consciousness. He does not encounter sick or disabled people on his doorstep, as was once the case, and still happens in societies in which sick people are not hospitalized because of cultural or economic reasons. In his childhood, when he contracted some temporary disease, he was immediately given medication that promptly and efficiently removed any possibility of experiencing pain or suffering. For years, he has assimilated the information that regularly inundates the media regarding newly discovered medications and cures that are conquering diseases. He lives in an environment that worships youth and "the culture of the body" and sincerely hopes that the relentless progress of science will succeed in eliminating illness and old age – and possibly death itself – before it is his turn to meet these shadows from the dark past of humanity.

The moment of realization, therefore, exposes the person to an intensity of emotion that he is not accustomed to in his everyday life. He rails against the injustice – after all, the illness has caught him at the most inappropriate time, and more than that, why him? – especially if he has been meticulous about his diet and his physical fitness and has eschewed the vices of tobacco and alcohol. However, his main feeling is fear. He is afraid of the suffering and of the loss of the freedom to do whatever he feels like doing. Mostly, he is afraid of death, of the final annihilation.

Things were different in the past. Even today, in traditional societies on the fringe of modern culture, it is possible to feel that illness and even death are part of life. Until only eighty or a hundred years ago, this was the reality – even in the most advanced societies of the time, in the heart of the European and Western culture. The most obvious difference between the beginning of the twentieth century and today is evident in the tremendous advancement in the knowledge and technology at humankind's disposal; this is particularly true of the field of medicine. All of the terrible epidemics that ripped people's lives apart without their being able to do anything to defend themselves against them have disappeared. We have only to remember the polio virus, which causes paralysis in children, that struck the entire world in the 1950s, and against which there was practically nothing to be done except wait and pray. Today, that same virus is the target of a global immunization campaign whose objective is to eliminate the disease entirely. This was already accomplished at the end of the 1970s with the smallpox virus, which threatened humankind for thousands of years.

The development of vaccines and antibiotics effected an enormous change in everything to do with viral and bacterial diseases – perhaps the greatest change ever in the field of medicine.

Today, with the decoding of the human genome, there is growing hope that we may be fortunate enough to see the rest of the human ailments, particularly cancer, going the same way as the infectious diseases and becoming subject – even partially – to human control. The experience of human power based on scientific progress is completely different than the previous feeling of helplessness in the face of disease that accompanied humankind, including physicians, for hundreds of years. One of the principal schools of thought in nineteenth century medicine stated that besides maintaining good conditions of hygiene and nutrition, medicine does not have the power to do anything to affect the course and final outcome of a disease. This school of thought was called "therapeutic nihilism" and it endowed the feeling of helplessness, mentioned above, with scientific grounds.

The change in the way humanity perceives its ability to withstand the forces of nature is linked to another change that took place over the last hundred years. It is essentially a spiritual change. The contemporary Western person, in an attempt to contemplate his life and find some kind of meaning in it, soon experiences loneliness closing in on him from all sides. This does not refer to the individual feeling of isolation and alienation experienced by a person who lives in a huge city among millions of other people with whom he has no human contact. It refers to the experience of "cosmic loneliness" in which the person does not identify any spiritual presence in his surroundings that can give his life purpose and meaning. Besides the chemical-biological process that is described in detail in the natural sciences, the modern human being is not able to utilize the power of his intellect in order to find a possible explanation for his existence. This chemical-biological process is random and devoid of any intention and purpose and is, of course, also indifferent to its consequences – to the human being himself. Until only one or two hundred years ago, the belief in God was still central to our ancestors' lives; they lived their lives in the knowledge that divine powers accompanied their every step. Today, in the best case, a totally abstract idea is all that remains of that belief. At most, the modern human being is prepared to acknowledge the existence of a superior force in nature that lacks direction and purpose, a force that is reflected in the harmony and beauty of the realms of nature, a force that by its very nature is indifferent to the fate of all creatures.

If the person's birth and life are meaningless, it is even more difficult for him to find a justification for suffering and illness. The irony of fate is that it is precisely when a person is afflicted by suffering and illness that he bestirs himself to seek some kind of meaning that will make it easier for him to endure the decree of fate. In those moments of his life, when the suffering causes him to be more sensitive to and aware of his thoughts and emotions, he encounters the full force of the extreme coldness of "cosmic loneliness". There is no cognizant, superior being in the whole wide world that has the power to help him. This experience of loneliness is what gives the modern human being courage; it is what sends him to fight the threatening forces of nature armed with nothing but his intelligence; it is what consecrates the war he has declared on illness and suffering.

In contrast, in the traditional societies of the past and to some extent in communities that preserve the past in the present, the person experiences himself as a part of an all-encompassing hierarchical system of spiritual beings rather than as a being that stands alone against a universe that is alienated and incomprehensible. The belief in God, from whom life and the meaning of life are derived, caused the surrounding world to appear less hostile, even though the person faced it helplessly. Even suffering and illness had a meaning and a purpose. They were perceived as a punishment for various sins of the individual or of the group to which he belonged. Sometimes they were actually perceived as a kind of trial by means of which the person could strengthen his soul and attain a higher level of perfection and of closeness to God.

When the contemporary human being faces the knowledge that he is ill, and questions concerning the meaning of the disease and the purpose of suffering arise in his soul, he has the possibility, of course, of going back and clinging to the old, traditional answers that proved themselves for eons. This solution is problematic because the answers that satisfied our ancestors were based on faith and not on knowledge. This is the same faith that exists even today in the traditional communities on the fringes of modern society. These communities are involved mainly in protecting their faith against any spark of independent thought that might undermine it. They consider the quest for truth, which so characterizes the modern person, to be forbidden. Ultimately, therefore, a person who seeks spiritual truth that does not deny the fact of his being an entity that is capable of independent thought, cannot be satisfied with the old answers. On the other hand, the principal trend of modern thought, which is expressed in the technological advancement and the medical progress of our times, does not relate to questions of meaning at all. Most of the modern philosophers have chosen to limit themselves entirely to questions for which they could find solutions within the physical world. Every question that aspires to investigate the meaning behind things necessarily touches on the metaphysical, that is, it strays from the limits set by the principal trend of modern thought.

The aspiration for a world without illnesses

Many people who are suffering from various diseases cling to the hope that in the near future, a new medication or treatment will be found to cure their illness. The more serious their illness, the more intensely they cling to the hope. Sometimes this hope actually materializes, because we really do live in an era in which science in general and medical research in particular make miracles happen all the time. Even so, in most cases, this hope is unfounded. The aspiration of science to eliminate all diseases as a part of humanity's aspiration to enjoy eternal life, free from all suffering, is unlikely to be realized. If it were a realistic aspiration, there would be no point in continuing to deal with the question of the meaning of disease, since it would anyway become irrelevant if diseases were eliminated.

However, when we look at the brief history of the efforts to eliminate diseases, we see that in parallel to the successes, there is the unexpected appearance of new diseases. One example is the occurrence of the first cases of AIDS in the Western world at the same time as the World Health Organization announced that the smallpox virus had been eliminated. Another example is the unofficial campaign throughout the developed world for early detection of fetuses with Down's syndrome and the deliberate termination of pregnancies in order to prevent the birth of these fetuses. During the same years, and in the same parts of the world in which the birth of children with Down's syndrome has almost entirely been prevented, there has been a steep increase in the number of children diagnosed as autistic during their first years of life. Is there a link between these disparate phenomena?

The question of the hope for a life without illness will be discussed later on. The two combinations that were devised by the history of humankind – the elimination of smallpox vs. the appearance of AIDS, and the decrease in the incidence of Down's syndrome vs. the increase in autism – have only been mentioned here in order to show that precisely when it seems that this hope is finally being realized in a certain field of medicine, new and incomprehensible diseases emerge from the depths of human existence and cancel out the technological achievements. Thus, at least for now, there is a call for continuing to deal with the question of the meaning of illness, both with reference to the evolution of humankind and with reference to the life of the individual. It would seem that diseases are going to be with us for a long time to come.

Anthroposophy and clarity of thought

In order to explore the meaning of disease, it is first necessary to clarify the meaning of life in general. It is impossible to understand the state of illness without understanding the state of health. In order to reach such an understanding, the knowledge of Anthroposophy, or spiritual science, will be employed here.

The inclusive world view that was initiated in the work of Rudolf Steiner at the beginning of the twentieth century in central Europe is called Anthroposophy (Greek: the wisdom of the human being). Rudolf Steiner was already well known as a philosopher and a researcher of natural science when he began to lecture to various audiences throughout Europe and open up new vistas before them. The material he presented was acquired from the direct experience of the supersensible worlds. According to Steiner, these supersensible worlds exist within and beyond the world of the senses and, together with it, constitute reality in its entirety. In other words, the world that is perceived by the person's senses is only a part of what really exists, and it is impossible to attain a comprehensive knowledge of reality if one ignores its supersensible components. Steiner also taught how one can attain supersensible experience and claimed that the path he was describing is open to anyone who chooses to walk along it[1]. In parallel, Steiner stressed that what is published as the fruit of Anthroposophy should be understandable to anyone with common sense. That means that even someone who does not choose the path of spiritual training can relate to the contents of Anthroposophy simply by devoting unbiased thought to them. The emphasis on clarity of thought as a prerequisite for supersensible revelation is what accords Anthroposophy its scientific quality, and this is the source of its other name – spiritual science. Alertness of consciousness, clarity of thought – these are qualities that are not usually held in high esteem by movements that deal with supersensible knowledge. This is evident in the scores of books that describe knowledge acquired, in states of clouded consciousness, by people who define themselves as channelers or mediums. However, what turns spiritual knowledge from something exotic into a force with true meaning in the twenty first century culture is precisely the accessibility to clear consciousness, to thinking consciousness. The relevance of Anthroposophy to life is evident in the fact that the spiritual research of Rudolf Steiner and his pupils is applied today in many fields such as education, agriculture, medicine, theater, art, architecture, economics and so on. In our case, anthroposophic research has made an indispensable contribution by making it possible to know the person's whole being with its spiritual and soul components. Without this knowledge, it would not be possible to achieve understanding of the question of illness and cure.

Many people who were raised in the modern culture shy away from emphasizing thinking. They tend to identify clear thinking with coldness of soul, alienation, and a cynical attitude toward life. People who feel this way are invited to continue reading in order to discover that the thoughts that flow from a spiritual view of the world are free of all the above mentioned traits.

The unique viewpoint of Anthroposophy enables the modern person to take advantage of the clear and free thinking that he has developed during the course of his evolution in order to uncover the spiritual background of the existential question of disease. Nowadays, many people in the Western culture who are facing questions of meaning turn to the ancient teachings of the East. These teachings, which originated in the tremendous spiritual revelations of past millennia, contain a great deal that is still relevant today. Since then, however, the human being has come a long way. While he has moved away from the spiritual world, he has acquired the capacity for independent observation and thinking. Thus, people who aspire to study the ancient texts and live by them encounter a limitation that is rather similar to the one that faces people who want to make a connection between Western religions and free thinking. Both Western religion and Eastern wisdom require that the believer or the pupil nullify his capacity for independent deliberation. On the other hand, Anthroposophy, which is not a religion, addresses the person's consciousness and invites him to think[2].

Illness and healing

In the following chapters, we will attempt to shed light on the manner in which an illness shapes the person's inner being. It is quite natural that the person's first reaction to the phenomenon of disease is an attempt to suppress it and prevent it from touching his life in any way. Fear is what causes him to banish thoughts about disease and death to the dark outer edges of his consciousness. Generally, later on, the person reaches the crucial moment in which he pulls himself together and begins to fight the disease. His aspiration to eradicate it from his own personal life is very similar to humanity's aspiration to eradicate all diseases. And just as humanity occasionally convinces itself that it is notching up another victory on the path to a life that is free of suffering, so does the individual. The last decades have witnessed the publication of many books and media items that describe people's victories over various diseases – cancer, in most cases. These publications attribute the victory to the spirit of the person who fell ill and recovered.

The reason for the increase in such publications lies first and foremost in the fact that there are more people who once had cancer living healthily among us. They recovered from various malignant diseases as a result of several factors. Most of them recovered from widespread diseases such as breast cancer or colon cancer because of the early detection of their disease at a stage in which it was still very localized. In this way, they could receive treatment – based mainly on the surgical excision of the tumor – that led to their recovery. Others recovered from rarer diseases for which modern medicine succeeded in finding medications that cure them, even if they were discovered at a more advanced stage.

What this means is that in most cases, the recovery is in no way linked to any kind of action taken by the person against the disease, but rather to the successful medical treatment he received. There would be no reason for mentioning this fact if it were not for the implied conclusion in books that describe the individual's victory over the disease. The conclusion that is not spelled out, but rather hinted at, is that anyone who does not recover from his disease evidently did not fight hard enough. He did not display sufficient determination in his battle against the disease. Perhaps he is less worthy in one way or another. Sick people who are exposed to these books frequently experience pangs of guilt for not succeeding in conquering their disease – after all, if they had only mustered their soul forces in the manner described in the book, they would have recovered.

Every physician – actually, every person – has the privilege of meeting people who withstand the tests of pain and suffering, of approaching death, of separation from their loved ones, heroically and courageously. Not only are these people not "defeated" by their illness, but they are the ones who really conquered fear and suffering. They are the ones who dared to meet pain and death with eyes wide open and learned about the meaning of illness from life itself. However, their triumph is not described anywhere. This book has been written as a testimony to the victories of many beloved people. In case any of the readers should mistakenly think that the life stories and the struggle of these people is described in these pages, I will have to disabuse them and say that this book contains only thoughts, suppositions and conclusions. However, thanks to what I learned from those modest heroes I had the privilege of knowing, and thanks to the gifts of courage and love they gave to those around them, this collection of thoughts could become a living reality for me. Of these women and men, some recovered, some live with their illness, and some departed from this world.

When a person seeks answers to questions about illness and cure, he has to learn to differentiate between the wheat and the chaff, between what is of value and what is useless.

Of all the people who have recovered from serious diseases thanks to modern medicine, there are some who did so in a manner that cannot be explained by medical knowledge, sometimes by the strength of their personality. Among all the general books about diseases and their cure, there are also some true pearls of wisdom and love. The only way a person can investigate the truth and understand his disease and how it is connected to his life is by means of clear and courageous thinking that enables him to separate the wheat from the chaff. The reader is therefore invited to read this book, too, with eyes wide open.

The human being

The fourfold nature of the human being

Modern natural sciences describe the human being as a gigantic weave of molecules that are continually coming together and separating again, and that duplicate and reproduce. The molecular depiction of the human being was made possible thanks to the development of the electron microscope, computers, and methods of identifying the components of the various molecules. It replaced the depiction of the human being that prevailed from approximately the mid-nineteenth century and perceived the human being as a collection of cells that make up various tissues. The cellular depiction of the human being was made possible by the invention and perfection of the optical microscope that constituted the spearhead of scientific research in those days. If we continue to go back in time, we reach the Renaissance when modern scientific research began with the dissection of corpses. Dissecting corpses constituted the first scientific breakthrough, revealing the structure of the internal organs of the human body and something about their function.

It is possible to see that the progress of human knowledge during the modern period is intimately linked to technological development. Every time a technological revolution occurred, it was followed by a revolution in the way the human being understood the world and himself. The great contemporary medical achievements can be attributed to technology and the ensuing knowledge. Another characteristic of modern scientific research from its inception until today is its focus on the dead body, the body that is devoid of life. The technology that led to the great achievements had and still has its limits. It can observe and investigate the dead body, the dead tissue, the various molecules after they have undergone some kind of freezing or stabilizing procedures that strip the life from them. The vast majority of modern scientific and medical knowledge has been garnered from the study and research of the dead organism. The modern natural sciences are based on an assumption that is self-evident to them – namely, that the laws that dominate the mineral world outside of the human being also dominate the processes that occur within the living organism. This assumption stops being self-evident when we notice the fact that the natural sciences have never investigated the processes of the living organism, but rather only the cadaver and its various components. Physics, the older sister of the natural sciences, knows that nothing but processes of breaking down and destruction can take place in lifeless matter. A process of organization or building can only occur as a result of an effect that works upon physical matter from the outside. Physical-mineral matter in itself is subject to the control of processes of breaking down and decomposition, as can indeed be seen in any organism from the moment life leaves it – in the human organism as well as in plant and animal organisms.

If this is the case, how do processes of growth and

development take place in the organism? How is life possible at all? As we have just said, processes of development, formation, growth and healing that occur in the living organism cannot stem from physical-mineral matter, but rather penetrate it from the outside. The system of laws that dominate the manifold phenomena of life in any organism, in their infinite complexity and in the wonderful coordination between them, stem from a higher principle that infuses physical matter with life. This principle can be called "the life body". Every organism that belongs to the plant or animal kingdoms has such a body. Only when it departs is the physical body subjected to the processes of breakdown and decomposition that dominate the mineral kingdom. The life body is not made of physical matter, however delicate, but rather from supersensible forces. One can have a direct experience of the life forces that comprise the life body of a particular organism by developing supersensible vision. In literature, one can find descriptions of life forces under various names. As an example one can mention the works of Goethe, the poet and writer who was also a prolific and very non-conservative researcher of nature. Goethe made important botanical discoveries as a result of his supersensible experience of the plant's life body, which he called "the archetypal plant". He maintained that the entire range of forms of the plant develops from one fundamental structure – the leaf. The laws that govern the development of the different forms of the plant world, as Goethe described it, are the laws of the life forces. Today, too, two hundred years later, the discovery of the development of the host of plant forms from the basic leaf form is still a fundamental hypothesis of botany. The supersensible experience at the basis of this discovery has long been forgotten.

Rudolf Steiner describes in great detail the requisite training for anyone who aspires to have a direct supersensible experience of the life body of the human being or the plant. As mentioned previously, Anthroposophy also enables people to attain a certain knowledge and understanding of the life forces through regular thinking. The present discussion does indeed address the reader's thinking, but it is narrow in scope. The aim of the thumbnail description of the life body and of the human being is only to permit the continuation of the discussion of the question of illness and cure. In the following chapters, too, several layers will be added to the description of the human being, but anyone who aspires to know more about the life body and the wealth of life forces and their diverse qualities should consult one of the fundamental books about Anthroposophy[3].

The life body exists in plants, animals and human beings. It varies greatly between one organism and the next, just as the physical bodies of various creatures are different from one another. All of the qualities that characterize a certain plant stem from its life body, but this is not true of animals. In the latter, there are functions such as sensation and movement that do not occur in plants, if we ignore several exceptions, such as carnivorous plants, for instance. A sensation of an external stimulus resulting in a deliberate approaching or retreating movement are the functions that appear in all of the organisms that belong to the animal kingdom – again with several exceptions, such as corals. The capacities for sensation, for the inner processing of the sensation, and for an appropriate reaction to what has been perceived by the senses, are qualities that attest to some kind of consciousness and to an active relation of the organism to its surroundings. The element that differentiates between the plant and the animal and contains these qualities we will call the "soul body". The soul body is also accessible to direct spiritual experience, and it exists both in animals and in human beings, albeit in a different form.

In human beings, it is not simply a matter of attraction, repulsion and a limited number of recurrent behavior patterns, as is the case in animals of a particular species. In human beings, there is an infinite range of behaviors that are not directly dictated by the sensory stimulus, but rather are dependent on the countless different emotions and considerations that arise in the human soul. A cat can only hunt a mouse, while a person has many possible choices. He can try to catch the mouse – even though he does so more clumsily than a cat; he can also chase it outside or even live with it; and he can jump onto a chair and scream. The cat's reaction is instinctive. It is dictated by its feline soul body that does not have the capability of choosing among different behaviors. In the human being, the soul body is subordinate to a higher element that grants his sensations and reactions an individual dimension. The person is not limited to an instinctive reaction of attraction or repulsion, but rather contains a whole inner world of emotions, desires and thoughts, which is also capable of self-awareness. The element that is unique to the human being, that develops an entire soul life on the basis of the soul body, will be called the person's "I", because of its individual quality that changes from person to person. Do not confuse what is called "I" here with what various schools of psychology call "I" or "ego".

The "I" is the human being's spiritual center. It makes every person an individual, a unique being among the various kingdoms of nature, a being that has the ability to affect the course of its life and give it a different character than the life of any other person. The unique course of the human being's life is his biography, to which we will return later on. Meanwhile, it is a good idea to find out how the person's supersensible components – that is, the life body, the soul body and the "I" – penetrate the physical body[4].

The four elements and the constitution of the human being

We have described the way the natural sciences currently perceive the human being – namely, as a collection of molecules. This perception is alien to the person's everyday experience. In his everyday consciousness, he perceives his body as a structure of substances that are solid to some extent or other and constitute his various body parts. The picture of the human being that is presented in anatomy lessons in medical schools also resembles the "solid" one more than it does the molecular one, despite the common knowledge that the human body contains more liquid than solid.

The body contains dozens of different fluid systems that are created from one another, separate and merge once again; for instance, the circulatory system with its subdivisions into the general circulatory system and the pulmonary circulatory system, into arterial and venous blood. Other fluids include intracellular fluid, extracellular fluid, lymph, gall, spinal fluid, urine, tears, perspiration, the secretions of the various glands, lubrication fluids in the various joints and so on. The blood is perhaps the only fluid that is perceived as a real tissue, as an inseparable part of the body. The rest are perceived as appendages, as bodily secretions, and not as actual components. However, the solid structure of the body is an illusion. Even the hard tissue of the bones of the skeleton is not something fixed and unchanging, but rather goes on breaking down and regenerating throughout the person's life. Of course, the rest of the tissues are also constantly being replaced and regenerating. Even if certain cells, such as in the nervous system, do not regenerate, their molecular components are still in a process of constant replacement.

While the bodily fluids are replaced at a faster rate than the solid substance, the rate alone does not make them into a less important component of the human organism. This observation opens the door to the understanding that in addition to his solid body, the person also has a fluid body. The fluid body is no less complex and no less structured than the solid body. It too has its laws of form and structure, which even take precedence over those of the solid structures. Suffice it to say that in the human fetus, the primary blood components are formed, and then the blood vessels are gradually formed around them. In other words, the blood fluid induces the vessel to be created around it. There are many more examples of the fact that the solid structures of the body are actually created from the fluid medium. Why should we dwell on this topic here? Because the person's metaphysical life body penetrates his physical body via the fluid element. It shapes the physical body, maintains the harmony within it and constantly cures it of the negative influences in its surroundings, via the fluid body.

The physical body also contains air. Air is no longer perceived as a part of the body from any point of view whatsoever. The length of time necessary to replace the gaseous component of the human body is extremely brief, even in comparison to the bodily fluids. There is in fact no barrier between the air inside the body and the air outside it. And even so, the study of the circulation of air in the body proves to be beneficial. We can begin from the entry point of air to the body – the nose and mouth, then via the trachea and the bronchial tubes to the lungs. We will see how part of the air, especially the oxygen, permeates the blood. By means of the blood and via the heart, the air reaches all the tissues in the body, where energy is produced. The by-product of this process, carbon dioxide, is collected from the entire body by the venous blood and reaches the lungs via the heart. From the lungs, most of it is exhaled. The energy or mobility of the body, which is one of the main expressions of the soul body, is closely linked to the respiratory process. Sensation, the second main property of the soul body, is also closely linked to the air in the body. All the sensory organs are surrounded by air: the entire skin is surrounded by atmospheric air; the eyes and the nose are surrounded by the facial cavities (the sinuses), which contain air in their normal state; the middle ear, which houses the auditory bones, is also an air cavity. We can generalize and say that if there is no air, there is no sensation. Thus, for instance, when fluid accumulates in a child's middle ear, his hearing is dulled. Alternatively, when air accumulates in the intestines, whose function is normally unconscious, we experience an unpleasant sensation. Even if we do not call it a body, the air in the organism still creates a defined structure that is the physical carrier of the motor and sensory functions of the soul body.

Whoever is familiar with the four elements that comprise the world in the ancient traditions of knowledge knows that after the solid or earth, fluid or water and gas or air, comes warmth or fire. Warmth is the vehicle of the "I", of the spiritual component of the human being. We will not go into this topic in depth either, but will content ourselves with mentioning a few contexts. All creatures are limited to life in a certain climate, to a certain range of temperatures. The ones that have fur survive in cold climates while those that can cool their bodies can tolerate hot climates. The human being is the only creature that can adapt the surrounding temperature to his needs. He does not have fur, but he controls fire – the element of warmth.

When body temperature is measured, we notice that it changes according to the hours of the day. Generally, it is low in the morning and rises by about half a degree or more during the day until it peaks in the evening. Then it decreases, and the whole cycle begins again. The rhythm of the day is the rhythm of the person's activity and actually the rhythm of the "I". The "I" is present in the body during the day and gradually raises the body temperature. In the evening, the person feels tired and needs to sleep. In parallel, his body temperature begins to decrease. During sleep, the "I" as well as the soul body detach themselves from the two lower bodies, the physical body and the life body, and body temperature continues to decrease. The rise in temperature is a physical expression of the activity of the "I" and the decrease in temperature is an expression of its withdrawal. A similar thing occurs during an illness with fever, in which the human individuality – the "I" – activates the immune system and produces fever. The high temperature reflects the increase in the extent to which the "I" grasps on to the human organism in reaction to the penetration of foreign elements such as bacteria or viruses. The heat works, both directly and by intensifying other mechanisms of the immune system, toward expelling the foreign element[5].

Waking and sleeping

In the complete picture of the human being described above, four components are combined. The physical body, in spite of the current cultural tendency to view it as the most important, is actually the end of the human process. It is constructed out of the substances of the surrounding physical world by means of the formative forces of the life body. The forces that create the life body do not spring from nowhere, either. They are gathered from the enormous ocean of life forces, which surrounds and penetrates the physical world. The principle that gathers the life forces from the general reservoir and creates the separate life body is the person's spiritual and soul nucleus – the "I" and the soul body. Those are the person's "higher bodies", which incarnate inside the outer sheaths of the physical substance and the life forces from the infinite world of the spirit.

The daily rhythm of waking and sleeping helps us

understand the relations between the bodies. The situation in which the higher bodies penetrate the lower bodies is the situation that is characterized by the person's waking consciousness during the day. During the day, the person accumulates impressions and influences from his surroundings. These operate in his entire being, from his physical body to the "I". After a period of activity in the physical world, the higher bodies need a break, a possibility to renew and refresh themselves by detaching themselves from the world of the senses and returning to the worlds of the soul and the spirit from which they originate. The higher bodies' need for a temporary detachment from the physical world is reflected in the feeling of tiredness, which is followed by sleep. During sleep, the person's lower bodies – the physical body and the life body – are in bed. The soul body, which has detached itself from them, stays in a sphere of soul forces and soul beings from which it draws new forces. The "I" is located in the spiritual world, and it too is nourished there by spiritual forces that enable it to go through another day of activity on the earth. During sleep, sleep consciousness prevails: the person does not move from his place, he does not sense his surroundings, and he is not aware of himself. This consciousness can be reminiscent of other beings that have a physical body and a life body that are not connected to higher bodies. Those are the beings of the plant kingdom. During sleep, when partial contact between the life body and the soul body is established, a state of consciousness somewhere between waking consciousness and sleep consciousness occurs: the dream. Dream consciousness also has a parallel in nature, and that is animal consciousness. The consciousness of the lower animals is very different than that of the higher animals. In the former, it is nearer to plant consciousness, and in the latter, it is nearer to waking consciousness – but without the human capacity for self-awareness.

Every morning, the "I" and the soul body bring fresh spiritual pictures with them from the higher worlds, and these act as a formative and constructive force on the lower bodies. However, during life, the physical and soul influences to which the person is exposed gradually cause the body to lose its power of renewal. The body of an adult, the life body too, is very rigid in comparison to the body of a young person. The aging body slowly moves away from the spiritual archetypes, various tissues and organs become calcified or atrophied, and the time when the physical body and the life body can no longer serve as a vehicle for the spirit approaches. Now sleep no longer affords the opportunity for regeneration, because the spiritual images cannot penetrate the hardened organs of the body. The end of the person's life on earth arrives. There is a similarity between death and sleep: in both of them there is a separation between the person's bodies, and in both of them the flow of the person's waking consciousness is interrupted. However, we perceive death to be absolute and eternal, while sleep is transient[6].

Spirit and soul come first

Anything that is found on the two sides of life, before birth or conception and after death, is off-limits to modern thinking. The present discussion exceeds the accepted limits and enters unknown realms. This requires reading that is different than ordinary reading, which is suitable for contents that are taken from everyday experience. Even the ideas that have been presented thus far required more than just pleasant reading in order for them to be deeply absorbed, but now the reader must be even more active, since the author's ability to help is limited.

When spiritual realities are discussed, even if they are explained in several different ways and demonstrated by the use of many examples, they can only be internalized by the reader if he musters all of his soul forces in order to grasp them. It is possible to compare spiritual truth to a goldfish in a pond that the person creates for it in his soul. The goldfish can exist in the person's soul only because he builds a pond for it and ensures that the water is clear. Another person can perhaps enjoy the description of the fish, but in order to see it with his own eyes, he also has to make an effort and create a pool of fresh water for it. He can do this, for instance, if he turns his gaze inward to his soul and conducts a small independent study.

The concept "soul" means the total of human experience. By means of the sensory organs, the person receives information about his surroundings and about himself. The process of receiving information is a process that involves the physical body, the life body and the soul body. This bodily process goes hand in hand with another process in which the person becomes aware of the sensory information that flows to him from all over. The second process occurs between the bodies on the one hand and the "I" on the other, and it is a process of soul. The soul is created and functions at the meeting point of the "I" with the three bodies. On the soul platform, the sensory information is revealed, along with the feelings that are compatible with it. The soul reacts sympathetically to some of the phenomena that are perceived by the senses, while it reacts with antipathy to others. Not coincidentally, this is reminiscent of the nature of the soul body, which moves between the poles of attraction and repulsion, of coming closer and pulling away. Sympathy and antipathy develop into the full range of feelings, and all of these together comprise the middle sphere of the soul. The feeling sphere is the semi-conscious sphere of the soul. The person may well experience his feelings very intensely, but is generally not aware of their source or consequences. The more conscious sphere is the thinking sphere. This sphere can be penetrated with full consciousness. Those are the two soul spheres that the reader is invited to contemplate. We will just mention that the human soul has another sphere, which is even less conscious than the sphere of feeling, and that is the sphere of the will. The will is the force in our soul that operates from the inside outward, to the surrounding world. As we will see later on, the person's motives for actions in the world do not reach his consciousness. In general, the person just thinks that he knows what motivates him to perform certain actions.

When the person looks into his own soul while at the same time remaining alert, he himself becomes a researcher. In this way, the reader can put what is written here to the test of his personal experience. While engaging in this inner contemplation, the reader must ensure that he maintains his concentration, since the mental contents that come toward him simply invite him to float with them and forget his original intention. It is also advisable to sit in surroundings that are not directly exposed to environmental stimuli. In this way, the possibility of being distracted from the contemplation by disturbances both from within and from without is reduced. During the contemplation, one should place a thought with spiritual content at the centre of one's consciousness and focus one's full attention on it. In this chapter, there are several thoughts suitable for this purpose. It is also possible to focus on a picture that describes or symbolizes spiritual reality. It is a good idea to avoid choosing pictures or thoughts that are emotionally charged, because they will disrupt the ability to contemplate, which requires peace of mind. It is important not to confuse the contemplation described here with various breathing or relaxation techniques. The state that is supposed to be attained by the person who practices this kind of contemplation is one of increased consciousness that focuses on a chosen image or thought. It is a state of intensified consciousness rather than a relaxed one.

One should repeat this exercise of intensive thinking a sufficient number of times, preferably for a short time every day. Frequently, months of practice and perseverance are needed. However, sooner or later, one becomes aware of subtle feelings that accompany the thought or the picture that is at the center of one's consciousness, and the thoughts themselves are revealed as beings that possess forces of growth and life. It is then that a new piece of knowledge, namely, that soul contents have an independent existence, is born in one's soul. Feelings and thoughts are not shadows that are cast by various physical objects, but rather real beings, even if their reality is not physical. Feelings and thoughts are beings that are made from the same "materials" as the ones that constitute the person's supersensible components. The person learns to know that his soul has an independent existence; in no way is it an appendage of his physical body, even if many of its contents have been accumulated by his physical senses[7].

The proposed contemplation is not the only way to learn about the independent existence of the soul and of the spirit. One can also put it to the test of thought.

If the soul were a product of the body, music would arouse similar feelings in similar people, or, in more current terms, people with a similar genetic makeup. We know that love of music depends mainly on education and not on the person's origins or genetic makeup. While the physical ear does have a role to play, as does the physical brain, the love of music exists as a soul content that goes beyond them. And what about music itself? It too has a non-material existence. A piece of music is a kind of idea that is first conceived by the composer's spirit, after which he "dresses" it in the sounds of various instruments and notes. Perhaps with a certain amount of effort and perhaps only at special moments, every music-lover can experience the spiritual nature of the piece of music through the sounds of the notes.

The music leads us to the Idea. One of Plato's bequests to Western culture was the knowledge that ideas, or thoughts, are spiritual beings that actually exist. This knowledge gradually disappeared over the years, until it was completely lost. The discussion that deals with the question of the existence of ideas has no relevancy whatsoever, according to the prevailing currents of modern thought, since it does not lead anywhere. Nevertheless, it is a good idea to clarify this question, because sometimes something good happens, and it can lead the person to the right path.

. The very fact that a contemporary person can take up the question of the ideas – which in itself is an idea – and grapple with it, attests to the fact of its independent existence. It is not a product of Plato's brain, but rather preceded him, just as it lasted for millennia after him. The pure idea, like music, is a spiritual being. A person who directs himself toward it can conceive it and put it in words or in notes that also enable people who do not have special talents and who live in distant places and at other times to become aware of it. The image of the idea as a spiritual being that is enveloped in a shroud of words in order to be realized in the world of the senses is very similar to the image of the human "I" that needs the different bodies in order to incarnate itself through them in the physical world.

Ideas are not the fruit of the brain, but rather precede the brain. Feelings precede the substances that are secreted by the nervous system – the neurotransmitters – and are not a result of them. This is also true for the spiritual and soul being of the human being as a whole, whose existence precedes physical existence.

Life beyond life and the law of karma

Clinical death experiences

It is only possible to reach a certain limit with everyday thinking. If the soul frees itself a little from the bonds of the materialistic perception of the world, it can, for instance, acknowledge the independent existence of thoughts. Through self-contemplation, it can see that even though its contents are influenced by its physical surroundings, they constitute first and foremost a part of the spiritual world that obeys laws of its own. It can also achieve the very general and vague knowledge that it had some kind of pre-birth existence and that the sum total of the experience it accumulated during its lifetime must be significant after physical death as well. Beyond these general pieces of knowledge, the power of everyday thought is not valid when we want to penetrate the secrets of life before birth and after death. For this reason, we have to turn to other modes of consciousness. For instance, it is possible to consult the reports of people who have undergone various supersensible experiences.

One type of description of supersensible reality that is fairly well known nowadays is that of people who experienced clinical death. These people describe their experiences when they were outside of their physical bodies. Many of these people's reports begin with a description of what is happening around their physical body – the efforts of the medical team to resuscitate them, for example. After this, some of them experience an event that changes their entire attitude toward life. They describe an encounter with a being that is radiating infinite light and love. This being shows them the events of their lives in a kind of huge living picture that is spread out before them. While they are in the vicinity of this being of light, they experience a deep feeling of consolation, and all they want to do is to stay near it, but they are sent back to their lives in the physical world because their day has not yet come. Whoever has undergone such an experience cannot go back and live in the same way as he lived before. He learns to devote his time to the truly important things, he gives of himself to the people around him, and he is no longer afraid of the day when he finally has to separate from his physical body.

The many clinical death experiences that have been described are different from one another in their intensity. Among those that have become renowned, the story of George Ritchie is particularly unique. Ritchie was an American soldier during World War II. He came down with acute pneumonia and died a clinical death – that is, he was freed from his physical body for a few minutes. While he was in a state of detachment from his physical body, he met the being of sublime light, which he recognised as the Christ. Ritchie's experience did not end with that. He was also taken on a journey to the world of the dead and saw what human souls experience after death. Ritchie was a very young man at the time, and his spiritual development did not end with his clinical death experience. Afterwards, he experienced other encounters that touched his soul deeply – he describes an encounter with a Holocaust survivor whose entire family had been slaughtered in front of his very eyes and despite that fact, had chosen to forgive the entire world, including the murderers. For the rest of his life, Ritchie tried to give a little of his experience of the light to other people. He worked as a psychiatrist and also wrote a book in which he described the experiences of people's souls after death, as he himself had learned directly years previously[8].

Among clinical death experiences, Ritchie's supersensible experience is extraordinary in its extent and its depth. In the introduction to this book, we mentioned that Anthroposophy describes a training method in which it is also possible to attain various supersensible experiences. Indeed, not every supersensible experience gives a comprehensive knowledge of life after death or before birth – in order to acquire such knowledge unusual abilities are required – but fortunately this knowledge has already been acquired and can be found in books. In ancient myths, we find descriptions of the person's journey after death, and less frequently before birth as well. The descriptions employ language and images in keeping with the period and culture in which they were written. There are also more modern descriptions from the twentieth century. Of those, we will use that of Rudolf Steiner, since it is the one that is most accurate and accessible to the critique of thought.

The world of the soul

Previously, we mentioned that the moment of death arrives when the physical body and the life body have worn out to such an extent that the higher bodies are no longer able to experience the world through them. The first tie that is broken is the one between the physical body and the other members of the human being. From this moment on, the physical body is ruled by the laws of the external world, which are reflected in the process of breakdown and decay. The human being, that is the "I" and the soul body, loses his ability to perceive the world of the senses through his physical sense organs, and he gains a completely different experience. The higher bodies, which previously resided in the physical body and experienced the physical world, now experience the life body that has freed itself from the physical body and surrounds them on all sides. Instead of seeing the physical world through physical eyes, they now see, by a supersensible perception, the life body that is all around them. Memory pictures that the person has accumulated throughout his life are stored in the human life body. Now they are spread in front of the human being in a kind of vast panorama that contains all of his experiences and deeds. This is the same picture that is described by people who have had a clinical death experience, but more complete and detailed. The human being sees the large life picture for about three days, until his life body is shed, and it too turns into a corpse and begins its process of breakdown in the expanses of the cosmic ocean of life forces. This period of time can be longer in a person who dies young, as his life body is still in the powerful grasp of the higher bodies.

Now the soul-spiritual being remains, surrounded by the world of the soul, and it has to find its way in this new reality. This is not the place to describe the different spheres of the worlds of the soul and of the spirit. We will just mention what is necessary for the furthering of our discussion[9]. The human being finds it difficult to become acclimatized to the world of the soul because it is in the clutches of the consequences of its actions on earth. In order to continue along its path in the spiritual world, it has to learn to know the true meaning of its deeds, words, feelings and thoughts. For a period of time that can continue for about a third of the lifetime it has just terminated in the physical world, the human being goes through what is called Hell or Heaven in the Judeo-Christian tradition.

In terms of spiritual science, Hell consists of the lower spheres of the world of the soul in which the human being meets up with his "sins". He burns in the fire of all the desires he did not overcome during his lifetime. Now, without a physical body, he is deprived of the possibility of fulfilling them. He also experiences the hurt he inflicted on others during his life. He experiences the pain he caused and the destructive consequences of his actions, which are now directed at him.

Heaven is the name given to the following spheres of the world of the soul. They are, in a certain sense, the continuation of Hell. Here the human being meets up with other deeds he did on earth, deeds that did not cause direct pain and suffering, but he has to separate himself from them as well in order to continue along his path. Here he meets the consequences of actions that were the result of his good intentions, but they lacked the recognition of the spiritual meaning of things. For instance, if a person was consciously a humanist and put his heart and soul into education, but the influence he exerted on young people was essentially materialistic, it means that it was devoid of awareness of the spirit. In these spheres of the world of the soul, the human being comes to realize that the foundations of his world view and thoughts and feelings often concealed egoistic or materialistic impulses. Only after the human being separates himself from what does not belong to his spiritual "I" is the path to his true home in the higher world of the spirit open before him.

Human development and the spiritual world

At this stage, after what has already been described and before continuing along the spiritual path of the human being , the fundamental question of purpose arises in all its acuteness. Why must the soul purify itself and become aware of the consequences of its actions in the world? Is it so that it can live for eternity in the company of its own kind, with the righteous or the sinners, in Heaven or Hell? The overt and familiar traditions of the Western religions do not provide a satisfactory answer to the question of purpose and meaning. In the West, the fragments of ancient knowledge about repeated lives on earth were kept secret by followers of the various mystery schools. Conversely, in the East, the knowledge of reincarnation and the law of destiny was overt, but thousands of years have passed since this knowledge was given to human beings in a direct spiritual revelation. As a result, it has moved far away from its live spiritual source and has become a dead tradition that also finds it difficult to answer contemporary questions.

In some of his basic books on Anthroposophy[10], Rudolf Steiner provides a broad description of the development of humankind and of the earth – the planet where humankind resides together with the kingdoms of nature. The subject of evolution is as broad and as deep as the sea, and whoever wishes to see the whole picture is advised to consult these books. Here we can only relate to the development of the individual, which is a small building block in the great development of humankind in general. Going back to the question of the purpose of existence, the one and only answer to it is human development. It is the objective of everything that the human being experiences both during his life and after his death, as we will see in the following pages.

Evolution does not only belong to the era when dinosaurs roamed the earth or to the places in which the new race of people – *Homo sapiens*, the thinking person – fought with his Neanderthal predecessors for hunting grounds. It is happening here and now, both the evolution of humankind and of the entire earth. Once, evolution was affected mainly by cosmic events such as the Ice Age, floods, and continental shifts. Today, the engine of evolution is humankind, who causes changes in climate, the extinction of plant and animal species, and other phenomena as a result of his uncaring attitude toward the consequences of his actions. Among the creatures most affected by his actions is first and foremost the human being himself. The contemporary person is different from the person that lived a millennium ago; he is even different from his grandfather who preceded him by fifty years. His everyday experience is different because, among other things, he is surrounded by technologies that separate him from the direct experience of nature. His height and weight are different and the diseases he contracts are different. He has a different view of the world and of himself. He thinks, feels and acts differently.

The current of evolution flows ceaselessly and in our era, its flow is becoming even stronger. The great current is made up of small droplets, of the development processes of the individual human beings. This development takes place in repeated lives on earth. During his life, the person accumulates many experiences, and after his death, he experiences them once again, both in the vast panorama of life that is spread out in his life body that is freed from his physical body, and in the world of the soul where he "relives" the consequences of his actions. When he encounters the true fruits of his actions, thoughts and feelings – this time from the spiritual point of view rather than the subjective point of view from which he observed his surroundings throughout his lifetime in his physical body – then the aspiration to set things right is born in his spiritual "I". He aspires to do good where previously he did harm, and to help the people he hurt. He can accomplish the aims he sets for himself by change and self-development. In the world of the spirit, the human being acquires an awareness of his weaknesses. However, overcoming his weaknesses cannot happen in the world of the spirit, but rather only in the physical world. Thus, the sojourn in the world of the spirit leads to the birth of the force that makes the human being incarnate once again in a physical body, and he does this in the presence of the particular souls whose destinies are intertwined with his. In the world of the spirit, the human being is accompanied by those human beings he met during his life on earth, as well as by more developed spiritual beings that do not incarnate in the physical world. These are the beings that are called angels or even gods in the various traditions, and they are the ones who devise the circumstances of the human being's next life on earth. The human being chooses the circumstances of his life, his place of birth and his parents, his physical properties, and to a certain extent, his diseases. He chooses the people he will meet during his life and what he must do for them. The higher beings are the ones who help the person attempt to realize everything his spiritual being aspires to achieve.

In the spiritual world, in addition to the beings that are linked to his individual destiny, the human being can meet the higher beings that are responsible for the development of the different nations and of humankind in general. In accordance with the degree of his development, he can join up with general human missions and serve them as well, in addition to the missions of his individual destiny.

Now the downward journey to the next life in the physical world begins. The spiritual "I" gathers the soul body from around him in the world of the soul. If the human soul in his previous life was permeated with spiritual striving, then a larger part of the old soul body is preserved and can serve as a basis for the new one. Then the human being continues his descent into the ocean of life forces. With the help of the higher spiritual beings, he forms his life body from it. The new life body is also constructed according to the functions it has to perform.

Moreover, it is the life body that determines whether the human being will be a man or a woman in his next life, among other things.

The womb in which the fetus develops is a special organ that enables the formative forces from the surrounding worlds to act within it. The person's spiritual being is the one that operates in the womb and engenders the growth of the fetus in it. To this end, it must make use of the "materials" it has at its disposal – the hereditary forces of the parents. In fact, it is mainly hereditary forces that are reflected in the physical fetus. Only after the birth does the "I" begin to operate in the infant's body in order to match what he has received from the stream of heredity to his needs. The purpose of the "I" is to enable the child's physical body, life body and soul body to develop the necessary forces so that in the future it can accomplish the individual tasks that its being took upon itself in the world of the spirit. We have already mentioned that the "I" operates physically by means of warmth. For this reason, children's diseases that are accompanied by a high fever are extremely valuable moments for the "I", which is aspiring to penetrate the physical body that has emerged from the stream of heredity and shape it in its own image.

Up until now, two main influences that shape the person have been mentioned. The first is the hereditary forces – it must be remembered that the human being chooses his parents and of course also his hereditary characteristics while still in the spiritual world. The second is the formative action of the "I" that gradually penetrates the bodies during the years of childhood and youth. There is a third type of influence: the events that the person experiences during the course of his life. These, too, originate in the spiritual "I", which continues to be linked to the world of the spirit and returns to it every night in order to re-encounter the pictures that shape its destiny. Between birth and death, the person has to meet the people who are connected to him from his previous life. He also has to go through difficult tests by means of which he will acquire the strength to cope with his life tasks. The sum total of the influences that are exerted on the person via his parents, via the formative forces of his spiritual being and via the events of his life, constitutes his biography. The biography is therefore the full expression of the person's spiritual being in the world of the senses.

The law of karma

Karma is the name of the spiritual law that regulates and shapes the person's present life according to the results of his previous lives on earth[11]. The word, which is thousands of years old, is taken from Sanskrit, and its literal meaning is action or consequence. Actually, karma is a spiritual reality that controls the person's destiny, but also contains the element of human choice between good and evil, that is, his ability to influence and change his own karma and that of the people around him. The difficulty in comprehending karma stems from its being a concept that is taken from the world of the spirit and translated into a language that is meant to describe the time and space of our physical world. A few pages back, the question of purpose and meaning was asked, and the answer was: human development. The entire law of karma is at the service of individual and general development. The human being in the world of the spirit, between death and a new birth, recognizes his need for correction. By means of the law of karma, he summons into his next life on earth the circumstances that will enable him to fortify himself and overcome his weaknesses or help someone he hurt in the past. Of course, in his everyday consciousness, the person is not aware of the action of karma, which is concealed behind external circumstances or "chance" encounters along his path. The life circumstances by means of which the person is strengthened are always difficult. People who suffer from some kind of disability sometimes develop tremendous strength of will and achieve things they would probably never have achieved had they not been disabled. Thanks to their disability, which requires a constant struggle, the person's forces of will grow. It is impossible to deny outright the possibility that the karma that caused the disability was directed at the development of the will. People who suffer from severe disabilities and do not attain extraordinary achievements also develop a strength of will that will be revealed in full during their next life on earth.

Medicine today is investing many resources to locate genes that cause cancer, and in fact more and more such genes are being discovered. However, not all of the people whose genetic makeup includes a particular gene will fall ill with cancer. The accepted medical explanation for the fact that some of the people who carry the gene will become ill and some will not is that besides the genetic tendency, exposure to an external factor with a carcinogenic effect must also take place. Only then will the disease occur. The following example is meant to explain the phenomenon in question from the point of view of karma: A human being that is between death and a new birth takes upon himself a task that he has to accomplish in his next life at a certain age. When the time comes, the person does not manage to fulfil the task. Perhaps he succumbs to fear, or the effort involved is beyond his capabilities. This is where karma steps in and helps the person develop the forces he requires for his task, by having to cope with a disease – cancer, for instance. The potential for the disease already exists in the genetic makeup the human being took for himself when he chose his parents while still in the world of the spirit. However, only after the person proves unable to accomplish his objectives with his available forces does the disease actually emerge.

The law of karma is neither absolute nor one-dimensional. The karma of the past realizes itself and at the same time builds itself as the karma of the future. It can develop in many directions, depending on the action of the person himself and also on the interrelationship between the actions of different people. The person can help other people realize their karma, for instance by means of education, medical or psychological treatment, or love. The person can also disturb other people and even seriously sabotage the realization of their karma. The first example of this kind of negative influence is very clear: parents who abuse their children. As we mentioned, the person already chooses his parents in the world of the spirit. Parents' commitment to their children's well-being and good is one of the sacred fundamentals of human society. In spite of this, people sometimes use their children to satisfy violent or sexual urges. A child who has been abused by his parents will have a very hard time rehabilitating his life. If he is not fortunate to grow up among people who give him warmth and love and serve as a substitute for parents, there is every possibility that he too will abuse his children one day. Thus, not only is his karma not realized, but a "negative" karma is created that begets more negative karma in its turn.

The following example of sabotaging karma is less clear and is accompanied by a bitter controversy: abortion. In modern society, many women choose to abort their fetuses for all kinds of reasons. Sometimes the woman is too young and sometimes she is too old. Sometimes the relationship between her and her partner is unstable, or their economic situation is bad. Sometimes a prenatal examination arouses the suspicion of a fetal defect. Sometimes this is definite and not just a suspicion, such as in cases of fetuses with Down's syndrome. The human being chooses his parents while he is still in the world of the spirit, with spiritual consciousness and in conjunction with his own and their karma. Thanks to modern technology, the parents can refuse to allow the fetus to be born. The couple or the woman chooses to terminate the pregnancy from the point of view of what suits them, a point of view that is very limited relative to the spiritual consciousness that motivated the human being to realize himself precisely in that particular fetus. The result is a disturbance to the karma of both the being that wants to be born and the parents themselves. It is important to stress that abortions in and of themselves, like any other medical tool, are not invalid. Sometimes they are essential for saving lives. Even when there is no threat to the woman's life, her right to make such significant decisions regarding her life cannot be undermined. However, the ease with which abortions are used as a contraceptive device creates disorder in the karma of contemporary humanity.

Abused children, as well as children who are forced to be born to parents other than the ones they chose in the world of the spirit, and human beings who, because of abortions, cannot realize themselves with disabilities that will afford them the life of difficulty and development they chose, will grow up with a defect in their strength of will. Weakness of will is the end result of most disturbances to karma. A person with a damaged will finds it even more difficult to realize the objectives he has set for himself in the world of the spirit for his continued development. Weakness of will obliges his karma to present him with a disease or a disability that will enable him to strengthen himself. The disease may come during his present life, or perhaps in the next life, after an additional sojourn in the world of the spirit.

A person's deeds in previous earthly lives create the karma with which he comes here. This is a karma of the past that shapes the person's present life by means of the three paths previously described: heredity, the action of the spiritual "I" on the bodies, and the events that occur along his path. However, influences that do not stem directly from his karma are also at work in his life – for example, deeds and decisions of other people. The examples presented previously related to child abuse and abortion. More general occurrences, however, such as wars or epidemics, are often not connected to the past karma of an individual. The person is hurt in a war because he happens to be a member of a certain nation and takes part in the general karma of that nation. He is harmed by an epidemic because he lives at a certain period and takes part in the general karma of that period. The trials a person goes through that do not stem from the karma of his past, join together with the results of his actions to create the karma of the future.

We see that the general karma of a period or of a group of people influences the karma of the individual. The influence can also work in the opposite direction. The karma of certain individuals sometimes influences the fate of many millions of people. The influence of an individual on the collective is clear to anyone who studies history or reads the newspaper. And even so, what is ostensibly so clear from the physical point of view may be the opposite from the spiritual point of view. Those individuals who are involved in the destiny of millions are generally sent to fulfill their historic role by the spiritual beings that shape the karma of the nation or period. In other words, the general karma uses the individual, who is only occasionally aware of the spiritual source of his deeds, in order to realize itself through him.

Ancient teachings of the East

The term *karma* is loaded. Many people, both in the East and in the West, are exposed to literature that suggests various ways of understanding it. Some of the teachings dealing with karma lump humanity and the animal kingdom together in one package. According to them, a person who sins is liable to be reborn after his death in the form of an inferior animal – a mouse, for example. These interpretations of the law of karma stem from ancient spiritual revelations from the period of the development of the Indian culture many thousands of years ago[10]. It is important to mention that the Vedas, which constitute the most ancient surviving Indian literature, were written some five thousand years ago. Even then, Indian culture was already past its prime. At that time, human consciousness was completely different from that of our time. The ancient Indians experienced physical reality as a shadow, as something that lacked genuine existence. They called the physical world *maya* – an illusion. The spiritual world, on the other hand, was very real to them. They perceived it in pictures and symbols. The human being's supersensible bodies were also directly perceived by them. They saw the lusts that reside in the person's soul body, for instance, in the images of inferior animals or insects. The spiritual picture they saw when they contemplated a person in the grips of lust can be compared to the experience of the contemporary human being after death, when he resides in the lower spheres of the world of the soul – in Hell. Anyone who looks at the paintings of Hieronymus Bosch or Matthias Grunewald's painting, "The Temptations of St.

Anthony", can imagine the experience of the ancient Indians. For them, this was reality and not just a work of art hanging on the wall.

The ancient spiritual revelations were transmitted by word of mouth for thousands of years until they were written down. Even after they were written down, they continued to metamorphose. When a modern person reads these books without knowing that they were written by people with a completely different consciousness from his own, his chances of understanding the content of the spiritual revelation on which they are based are small. This is the reason why errors occur. The opinion that a human being can be reborn as an animal and an animal can be reborn as a human being is one of those errors.

The whole human being, as presented in the previous chapter, is centered around an individual spiritual nucleus – the "I". Karma is the principle that directs the development of this spiritual being between birth and death and between death and a new birth. In contrast, animals do not have an "I". The individual person is not comparable to the individual animal but rather to the entire biological species. The individual mouse does not have karma, but the mouse species does. This is true for lions and tigers as well. Every such biological group is borne by a spiritual being that is not incarnated in the individual physical animal but is rather connected to the entire group. This spiritual being, which is actually identical to the biological species, has a karma.

The karma of humanity is closely linked to the karma of animals. Humankind has been able to keep on developing, at the cost of sacrificing the animals that served him faithfully during the course of evolution. He used them for transportation and work in the fields, for the production of food and for food itself. The treatment they received in exchange was in many cases brutal exploitation, the most extreme example of which is today's industrial breeding of various animals. Humanity's debt to the animals is a debt that is engraved in its karma.

The understanding of karma and the future of humanity

The fabric of the law of karma is all-embracing. As mentioned previously, each person has his own karma, which is intertwined with the karma of many other people. He has karma from the past and he has karma that creates a future. Groups of people also have karma. These groups can be communities with blood ties such as a family, a tribe or a nation, but also communities that people choose, such as a commune, a professional association or a monastic order. The sum total of people who live in a particular era have a common karma – the karma of the era. Humanity, too, some of which now lives in the physical world and some in the world of the spirit, has karma. Animals have collective karma. The other kingdoms of nature have karma, too, which is part of the karma of the entire earth. And finally, the higher spiritual beings that are not incarnated in physical bodies, that guide the development of the individual and the earth, also obey the law that directs the development of the entire universe.

Karma is a law of cause and effect. No knowledgeable

person expects anything to come from nothing in everyday life. In contrast, when the scientists try to explain the evolution of the whole planet, they speak about randomness, probability, about the hand of chance that turns a certain gene into a success story or sends it to oblivion. If this scientific theory had remained within the precincts of the universities and research institutes, the history of the last two hundred years would have looked different. However, the Darwinian perception of the world spread from the field of the natural sciences and turned into one of the main factors that shaped the economic, social and spiritual life of humanity in the modern age. The Darwinian view of nature as a constant battlefield in which the survival of the strong entails the oppression of the weak nourished the brains of the Communist thinkers, and its twisted visage leered over the Nazis' shoulders as well. It is the justification and the pretext for the capitalistic lust for Mammon and for every egoistic action performed by a person or a group of people. This perception prevents the person from understanding that his own good is inseparable from that of his neighbors and of the earth and of the air around him. He cannot expect a better future while he eschews his responsibility for other nations, for dead rivers and polluted seas, for plants that are becoming extinct, for the industrial breeding of animals, for his neighbor across the street.

In order to attain a true understanding of the laws of karma, it is necessary to study them in depth. Reading Rudolf Steiner's lectures about karma is a good start. Gradually, the spiritual concepts change from abstract terms into real forces that operate in the soul. Then comes the stage in which the interest in karma ceases to be theoretical and the person sees his life and his relations with the environment in a new light. He begins to feel a growing responsibility toward what is happening in his immediate and distant surroundings. He experiences the hidden strings that bind his individual destiny to the destiny of the earth and all of its creatures. The spiritual world view, which is founded upon an understanding of karma, opens a door to a better future for humanity and for the whole of creation.

Illnesses

The development of the understanding of disease

For eons, human beings have tended to blame diseases mainly on external factors that are not a part of what they perceive as themselves. The ancient Greeks believed in the Moirai, the three goddesses of fate that spin the thread of the person's life, afflict him with troubles, and break the thread when his time on earth is up.

According to the principal view of the Jewish faith, diseases come from God. While it is also possible to find sources in Judaism that blame suffering on a person's bad deeds, there is always the opposite view of reality, of "the righteous suffer, the wicked thrive". This negates the direct link between the disease and suffering that afflict the person and the fact of his being a sinner. In the New Testament, on the other hand, there is sometimes a clear connection between the illnesses that afflict the person and his sins. Christ heals some of those who come to him by forgiving their sins. However, later on in Christianity, this connection between the person and his ailments was no longer obvious as it was in Christ's time.

In the eighteenth century, medicine still viewed the cause of diseases as an imbalance among the four basic fluids of the body. The roots of this view can be found in the writings of Hippocrates, who wrote the first medical texts in the West from spiritual knowledge that originated in the Greek mystery centers. The body fluids were perceived by Hippocrates as the conveyors of the life forces and not as dead mineral fluids. However, the physicians' ability to understand the spiritual knowledge presented by Hippocrates diminished over the generations, just like the ability to understand the ancient Indian texts. Ultimately, the "humoral" theory – the theory of the body fluids – became completely materialistic, did not succeed in explaining new discoveries, and fell victim to the pioneers of modern science and to bacteria.

Since the discovery of microorganisms through the microscope lens and until recently, they were thought to be the major causes of diseases. This medical approach, in contrast to the theory of fluids, succeeded in notching up real achievements in the cure of contagious diseases, thanks to the discovery of various types of antibiotics. Having said that, it is worth recalling that the first vaccine in the Western world, the vaccine against smallpox, began to be administered when the humoral theory was still in force and was also successfully explained by it. In recent decades, links between microorganisms and diseases that were not previously thought to be ordinary infectious diseases have been found, for instance viruses and certain types of cancer, or a bacterium that plays a role in the formation of gastric ulcers. Thanks to these discoveries, bacteria and viruses still have their place in modern disease research.

However, the leading school today in the study of diseases is the one that seeks the cause of diseases in the person's hereditary makeup – in his genes. Diseases that are caused by bacteria or viruses can cause great damage to one person and not affect another at all. This is also the case with cancerous diseases that are linked to certain viral infections; not everyone who is infected with the virus will develop the disease. The bacterium or virus may be identical, but different people will react to them differently. The reason for this is being sought in the genetic makeup. It is hoped that the action of the defective genes can be repaired, or that the action of the harmful genes can be neutralized, in this way reinforcing the person's resistance to disease.

We began the chapter with the claim that the human being has always tried to distance the causes of disease from himself, but both body fluids and genes are nonetheless part of him. Despite this fact, they are not part of his self-perception. They are alien to the person's soul, which experiences them as external to it. In this context, it is interesting to point out the similarity between the terms that are used in the modern theories of the source of diseases and those employed in modern computer technology. In the computer world, too, there are "viruses" that infect the computer and damage it. The way to defend oneself against them is by blocking loopholes in the computer program and reinforcing its ability to identify viruses and annihilating them – or, in other words, repairing its "genome" and its immunity against diseases. If a person wants an explanation for his disease from his physician, he generally receives a "technological" explanation that describes a process that resembles a mechanical, electrical or electronic mechanism. Even if the person is satisfied with this answer, after he has examined it with another physician or on the Internet, his soul is not satisfied at all. Despite the fact that there is a good deal of truth in all of the above mentioned theories, they remain alien to his soul. They have nothing to do with the existential question of the sick person.

Alongside the mainstream of medicine, there are also the "alternative" approaches, which blame the cause of illnesses on various "energies". Among these is magnetic or electromagnetic radiation, subterranean water currents and "negative" thinking. Other theories are based on factors such as a fungus called candida, tooth fillings that contain poisonous metals and many others. All these theories have two things in common: first is a particular element of truth that is found in most of the "alternative" theories as well as in all the theories that are used by conventional medicine. The second is that every one of them has groups of sworn supporters who would do anything to promote it without relating to its true importance in the least.

Evolution – Lucifer and Ahriman

Just like the human genome and the bacteria and viruses that attack people, diseases are a part of human evolution. Two different descriptions of evolution are presented in the form of two Creation stories in the Book of Genesis. The first story, which begins with the words, "In the beginning, God created the heaven and the earth", describes the evolution of the earth and of humankind from the physical point of view. If we focus on the order of the appearance of life on the face of the earth – without the astronomical and geological events – the biblical description largely fits the evolutionary theories of the natural sciences. First the plants develop. The development of animals begins in the ocean. After the marine creatures, the reptiles and the birds appear. Only on the next day, a new age, the animals appear – meaning mammals, and finally humankind.

The second Creation story is very different from the first. Initially, the creation of Adam is described, and only afterwards are the other kingdoms of nature created. God plants a garden and grows plants, and afterwards creates the animals and brings them to Adam so that he can give them their names. The significance of the name-giving, according to the commentators, is separation. Humankind separates the animal nature from himself – the cunning of the fox and the stubbornness of the mule. This separation enables him to develop unhindered by the single-sidedness that is characteristic of all animals. A person can choose not to be a fox or a mule, an ant or a cricket, that is, he can be free.

According to the second Creation story, humanity's ancient spiritual being, which had not yet been divided into male and female and had not yet separated into individual human beings, is the starting point for the entire evolutionary process. From this spiritual being evolution separates the animals, which materialize on the earth one after the other. The two Creation stories of the Book of Genesis are not contradictory, but rather complement each other. They describe exactly the same process from two different points of view. The second story is told from the spiritual point of view – the Creation process begins with the primordial spiritual being of humankind, from which all the creatures of the physical world gradually derive. The first story, in contrast, is told from the terrestrial point of view – the various plants and all the kingdoms of the animal world appear on the earth, from the lowest to the highest, until humankind appears as the crowning glory of the evolutionary process.

The discussion of the Creation stories is not directly related to the topic. It is presented here in order to show, albeit briefly, that the ancient texts contain a great deal of wisdom and extremely precious spiritual knowledge. From this point of view, the creation stories of Genesis are similar to all the ancient mythologies, which present rich pictorial descriptions of spiritual realities. The source of the ancient mythologies and of the writings of the different religions lies in the mysteries, in those places in which people who underwent special initiation were in direct contact with higher spiritual beings and received spiritual knowledge from them. The spiritual knowledge that resides in the ancient mythologies is imparted in pictures and not in abstract thoughts. The explanation for this comprises at least two layers. On the one hand, our ancient forefathers were incapable of the abstract thought to which we are so accustomed today – the development of and change in human consciousness even in a few hundred years has already been mentioned. On the other hand, the pictorial image is by nature flexible and varied, and is therefore more suited to describing the complex and multidimensional spiritual reality than abstract thought.

Today, too, anyone who wants to describe spiritual reality faithfully must use the tremendous pictures by means of which the world of the spirit is revealed to people who are spiritual seers. In other words, Anthroposophy also has a "mythology" that describes the spiritual beings that work on and influence human evolution. It would be possible to use abstract concepts to describe the various forces at work in the human soul that cause diseases, among other things. However, it is important to understand that those soul influences are the fruit of the workings of spiritual beings that express themselves not only in the person's soul, but also in his body and in his natural surroundings. The use of pictures from the anthroposophic "mythology" instead of abstract concepts opens the door to a living and genuine understanding of the forces that motivate human development. The pictures are symbolic but not imaginary. They represent spiritual beings that are completely real, beings that are more complex than our everyday thinking can conceive of.

Now we will use the continuation of the Creation story, the description of the temptation of Adam and Eve by the serpent in the Garden of Eden. The higher beings that lead evolution are the ones that are responsible for the creation of the human being in their image, that is, as a spiritual being. This young being was supposed to go through eons of slow and protected development, under the protection of the spiritual hierarchies, as Rudolf Steiner calls the higher beings. However, a glitch occurred in the celestial plan, or perhaps an unexpected step that was a part of the plan. Lucifer, as he is called in anthroposophic literature and in ancient occult writings, was also a higher spiritual being that fought against the divine leadership and aspired to extricate humankind from God's field of influence and induct him into his own service. To this end, Lucifer – he is the seducing serpent in Genesis – gave humankind the fruit of the tree of knowledge long before this was meant to happen. As a result, self-awareness began to emerge in the human soul body, which was already far along in its development, while his independent spiritual being, his "I", was still right at the beginning of its development. The young "I" was not yet capable of harnessing the new abilities of the soul body, and it began to lag behind it during the course of human evolution. After the Fall – the expulsion from the Garden of Eden – the human being began to experience himself as an individual being that was separate from the gods. He also began to develop his own wisdom, but, in parallel, the door to immoral action and egoistic deeds was opened to him.

The results of the Luciferic temptation were momentous: First, the possibility of sin was born. Divine morality no longer guided humanity, while human morality had just begun its development, which has not ended to this day. Second, the human being was expelled from the Garden of Eden; that is, he lost the feeling of the direct presence of God and came closer to the physical world. Here, in the physical world, he shifted even further away from the path traced for him by the spiritual hierarchies. The world of matter took hold of his consciousness increasingly strongly and caused him gradually to forget his spiritual source.

The influence of the world of matter, too, like any reality, stems from the action of spiritual beings. In the ancient Persian religion, Zarathustrianism, the entire world is perceived as a struggle between the god of light – Ahura

Mazda, and the ruler of the darkness – Ahriman. The being that attracts humankind to matter and darkens the light of the spirit in modern consciousness is the same being that has been identified by Zarathustra as a force that opposes the godhead and is called Ahriman[10].

The human being as a battlefield

Humanity's entire evolutionary development occurred in the tension between the influences of Lucifer and Ahriman. We have already mentioned the three forces of the soul: the conscious sphere of the soul is thought, the semi-conscious sphere is feeling, and the sphere that remains outside of the person's consciousness at his present level of development is the will. The will is a force of soul that enables the person to act and to do. The person's spiritual "I" operates through the will in order to realize his karma. It leads him to meet his karma every single day by means of new people or events, without his consciousness playing any part in it. However, not only the human "I" that cooperates with the higher beings that regulate the person's karma works through the will. Lucifer also does. The Luciferic influence, which resides in the soul body, introduces the egoistic element into the person's deeds in the world. Selfishness is the force that motivates many human deeds, some of which are actually intended to do good. In works of art or thought, for instance, there is a Luciferic element that aspires to give the person's soul pleasure. In the relations between people who are close, there is a Luciferic element that is expressed in the person's desire to be good to the people that are dear to him. Even the idealistic aspiration for the lofty and spiritual contains a Luciferic overtone that causes the person to link good with what is externally fair and pleasant to the eye and to deny the possibility that a higher spiritual element can also be expressed in the guise of ugliness. Of course, it must not be forgotten that human egoism is expressed first and foremost in a much more direct and blunt manner through evil, cruel and exploitative deeds.

From the other side, the Ahrimanic influence is at work on the person. From the historical point of view, the human being enters Ahriman's domain only after he has distanced himself from the protection of the spiritual hierarchies as a result of the Luciferic temptation. While it is possible to identify the powerful Luciferic element in the ancient cultures of the East, Ahriman is revealed at a later time, through the modern materialistic and technological culture of the West. The ancient Indians still experienced the spiritual beings as more real than their external physical manifestation that they called *maya*. At a later time, the direct perception of the spiritual beings gradually declined and the perception of the senses enveloped all human consciousness. The memory of the spiritual world shifted away, the great mythologies became folk stories, and even the religions became more and more intcllcctual. Judaism, which in its first millennium was a religion of ritual and commandments that were linked to an agricultural life, became a religion of study and thinking. In Christianity, the difference between Catholicism and later Protestantism is prominent. The Catholics believe that during mass, the bread and wine are turned into the actual flesh and blood of Christ, while the Protestants perceive the bread and wine more as symbols and not the real thing. The Protestant houses of worship are designed with an impressive simplicity that addresses human rationality, while the Catholic cathedrals, which preceded the Protestant houses of worship, are great works of art that affect the person's entire being. Lucifer is revealed in the human soul via the will, while Ahriman penetrates the human being via his thinking.

The materialistic tendency dominates all areas of life today: sciences, society, economics, industry, agriculture, and even religion. The Darwinian theory, which was mentioned previously, is an example of a way of materialistic thinking that denies the spirit and bases the development of the whole of nature on blind randomness. The way in which Darwinian thinking has insinuated itself into social and economic domains in the last two hundred years – there are Darwinian elements in communism and capitalism – attests to the power of Ahriman's influence on our world.

Cars, computers, washing machines, airplanes, antibiotics, operating rooms and intensive care units, efficient administration – these are the gifts of Ahriman. So is the person's inability to see other people as spiritual beings, the dependence he develops on material possessions, his aspiration to find in them security from the unknown, his lack of hope in a life devoid of meaning, and his fear of death.

Between the will that is implemented in the limbs and thinking that observes the world from the head up above, there is the middle sphere of the soul – the feelings. They can be attributed to the chest region where the heart and lungs are situated. The heart and lungs are in a state of perpetual rhythmic motion, expanding and contracting over and over again. Similarly, feelings shift between expansion and contraction, between sympathy and antipathy, between will and thinking. From the two poles, Lucifer and Ahriman work on the middle sphere with the aim of subjecting it, and thereby the person, to their domination. It is possible to differentiate between "warm" feelings, which are closer to the will and the Luciferic influence, and "cold" feelings, which tend toward thinking and the Ahrimanic influence. The anger that burns inside is an example of the first type. It generally has a personal tinge and stems from a feeling of insult that can be expressed in the words: "How can they do that to me?" Passion and joy are also warm emotional processes that are linked to the will.

From the other pole comes the bone-chilling fear that freezes people and makes them weak at the knees. Fear paralyzes movement, the action of the will; it is an example of an Ahrimanic domination of the middle sphere. Thriftiness and stinginess are Ahrimanic traits that indicate the cold considerations that overcome the urge for uncontrolled spending. The feeling of obligation that directs people to act in accordance with principles rather than to satisfy their desires also attests to the domination of the thinking pole in the person's soul.

Anyone who is accustomed to the clear dualistic division between good and evil or between God and Satan has to display mental flexibility in order to adapt to the pictures of Lucifer and Ahriman presented here. If, at the end of the description, it is still not clear to the reader whether they are good or bad, the description will have been successful at least from one point of view. Lucifer and Ahriman are spiritual beings that pull the human being in opposite directions. Human development toward freedom occurs between their spheres of influence. We can judge a person's deeds as good or bad, and even then we have to remember that the point of view of our judgment is blind with regard to the spiritual foundation of things.

The tension between the two poles, Lucifer in the will and Ahriman in thinking, conceals the right road that will lead the person to the gods once more – this time as a spiritual being that shapes its own destiny and the destiny of the kingdoms of nature for which it is responsible, with the help of the forces it has acquired during the course of its development.

What is illness?

A person lives his life until the end. When he reaches the world of the soul after leaving his physical body and life body, he experiences his life again but in reverse. He now faces the consequences of the deeds and actions he directed at the world and other people during his life on earth. In this way, he learns the weaknesses that overcame him over and over again, and knows with a certainty that is unlike anything he encountered in the life between birth and death what he has to correct. The higher beings of the spiritual world – those that shape the bodies that will serve him in his next life – come to his aid. It is not always possible to correct everything in one earthly life, and this is when karma from several incarnations accumulates. It is important to remember that every person alive today has accumulated a great deal of complicated karma during the course of many incarnations. This is one of the reasons why, in stark contrast to the past, when most people lived their entire lives in the same village, the lives of many people nowadays are so rich in new experiences.

In order to understand the mode of action of the karma via illnesses, it is a good idea to begin with relatively simple examples and then to progress further toward the complex diseases of our time. The first two examples are diseases that have accompanied humanity for thousands of years. While they are no longer a part of modern life in the rich and developed countries, they are still a part of the traditional and fairly simple lives that people lead in vast areas of the world. One of them, malaria, is one of the most widespread diseases in the world even today. The two examples are taken from a lecture series by Rudolf Steiner, which is indispensable for anyone who wants to learn about karma[11].

The first example concerns a person with a weak sense of self, a person whose actions are strongly influenced by his surroundings and who is hesitant in taking a stand or working toward the goals he set himself because of low self-esteem. After death, during his sojourn in the world of the soul, he becomes aware of the way he behaved and how he affected his surroundings prior to death. Then the profound desire to develop a strong sense of self during his next life on earth is aroused in him. He undertakes to seek out the circumstances that will help him succeed in strengthening his "I" forces. His spiritual being aspires to shape a soul body, a life body and a physical body for itself that will present it with the great difficulty that is necessary for it to develop the consciousness of its "I". Steiner says that a person like that will unconsciously search for an opportunity to contract cholera during his next life. Cholera creates the physical circumstances that present the spiritual "I" with the necessary resistance for the development of a strong earthly presence that will generally come to the fore only during the next earthly life. In other words, the weakness in one incarnation requires compensation during the course of the next incarnation, so that there will not be any weakness in the third incarnation. Sometimes, if the person recovers from the disease, the new quality is already manifest in that particular life. All that remains is to find out why it has to be cholera.

The opposite example is that of a person with too strong a sense of self, who went through life without understanding his surroundings or taking the people around him into consideration. When this human being is reborn after his sojourn in the world of the spirit, he will do so in places where he can contract malaria. The bodies of the person with malaria do not offer resistance to the "I" that penetrates them – on the contrary, they enable it to penetrate deeper and deeper into them and display ever decreasing resistance. By means of experiencing this extreme situation of penetration without resistance and without holding on, the "I" will develop the self-restraint that it aspired to achieve – either in that particular life or in the next.

Cholera is a bacterial disease that is transmitted through human excrement. The outbreaks of the disease occur through contaminated drinking water or crops. The bacteria damage the wall of the intestine and cause a massive loss of fluid in the form of very acute and watery diarrhea. If the disease is not treated by the administration of large quantities of liquids, it usually culminates in death from dehydration within a few hours or days. Through cholera, the "I" achieves the fierce resistance of the bodies that is necessary for reinforcing its sense of self. The resistance is linked to the process of dehydration that takes place in all the tissues of the physical body, especially the blood. The blood is the fluid into which the "I" penetrates to the greatest extent, with the help of warmth. Within a short time, the sick person's blood becomes thick and very concentrated. With a little imagination, it is almost possible to feel the great resistance the spiritual being experiences while attempting to go on penetrating the blood of the sick person.

Malaria is caused by a parasite that is transmitted through a mosquito bite. It enters the red blood cells and multiplies in them. After a period of a few days, all of the affected blood cells break down and release the new generation of parasites into the bloodstream. Once again, they penetrate new cells, and the cycle goes on. During the times when the parasites are released into the bloodstream, the person suffers from exhausting attacks of high fever and chills. The red blood cells contain hemoglobin that supplies oxygen to all of the body's life processes. As a result of the destruction of the cells, the blood becomes thinner and thinner. The disease can manifest itself mildly and remain with the person for years, or it can take on an acute form and cause a massive destruction of the blood cells in a short time, endangering the person's life. By thinning the blood, malaria gives the "I" the experience it was looking for. The

"I" tries in vain to strengthen its grip on the body, as evidenced by the attacks of fever, but because of the thinness of the blood, it only grasps liquid. The blood, which contains fewer blood cells, little hemoglobin and little iron, does not offer any resistance to the person's spiritual being, and does not provide it with a handhold. This is the experience that is necessary for restraining the person's sense of self.

What arises from these two examples has already been implied in the previous chapters. From the spiritual point of view, which is shared by the higher spiritual beings that lead the evolution of humanity, the beings that serve the development of the individual and the spiritual human "I" itself, the real disease is the weakness that is found in the human soul. What is experienced by the person in the physical world as a disease is the vehicle employed by his spiritual being in order to overcome his weaknesses. The person himself, who suffers from the disease that he contracted, is the one who chose the disease while at a higher level of consciousness during his sojourn in the world of the spirit prior to his birth.

This thought is liable to seem completely contrived to the person's everyday consciousness, but it is precisely people who have experienced a serious disease in their life who can identify with it to some extent. For these people, it is not an abstract thought, but rather an existential experience. They are frequently capable of identifying within their soul the true forces that were born inside them as a result of the disease.

Warm diseases and cold diseases

Human diseases can be roughly divided into "warm" diseases and "cold" diseases. "Warm" diseases – febrile illnesses – are those that are characterized by a rise in temperature following the activation of the immune system against a cause of disease such as a bacterium or a virus. "Warm" diseases appear significantly more in infants and children and less in adults. "Cold" diseases, which are more common in the latter, are diseases that stem from metabolic disorders such as higher fat or sugar levels, the formation of deposits in the organs, calcification and atrophy. Many diseases cannot be classified so simply; some of them begin as "warm" diseases and shift to a "cold" chronic stage, and some of them do the opposite.

As we have already mentioned, warmth is the element through which the human "I" strengthens its grip on the body. The effects of febrile illnesses will sometimes be felt immediately after the illness, and sometimes many years later. The short-term effects can be discerned by observant parents. Frequently, the fever erupts following a period of time in which the child does not find his place, whether this is in his body or in his surroundings. A change can occur as a result of the illness – for instance, acclimatizing to a new physical or social situation, or the disappearance of chronic weaknesses such as skin problems, a lack of appetite, recurrent infections or fears. The long-term effects of febrile illnesses are more difficult to identify. Various researchers have found a relatively low incidence of "cold" diseases of particular types in adults who came down with more febrile illnesses in their childhood[12]. The difficulty in such research stems from the very attempt to link two phenomena that are far from each other in time. These "cold" diseases, which include certain types of cancer, occurred in adults many years after the low-key or non-appearance of febrile illnesses during childhood. During the course of their lives, these people were exposed to many additional influences that were liable to cause diseases, and this explains the difficulty of isolating and assessing the importance of the effects from childhood on the adult. Despite the difficulties, there are studies today that link many phenomena in adults, ranging from obesity to various mental phenomena, to influences to which they were exposed in childhood.

On the soul level, the tremendous importance of childhood as the formative period in the person's life is undisputed, as anyone can confirm from personal experience. In spite of this, the long-term physical effects of childhood are a bone of contention, since public recognition of the existence of these effects would necessarily entail far-reaching changes in many areas that relate to infants on the one hand and to certain vested interests on the other. The link between feeding infants with substitutes for mother's milk and weight gain and other problems in adults, is a good example of a long-term physical effect that is not accorded the proper public attention. The same goes for the febrile illnesses. The recognition of the link between these diseases in children and the "cold" diseases in adults is likely to have immediate implications for very practical aspects of the health policy – for instance, the overwhelming tendency to immunize all children against every possible disease, including diseases that are not life-threatening, or diseases to which only certain populations are susceptible.

In order to find out what the spiritual significance of "warm" and "cold" diseases is, we will follow Rudolf Steiner and consider another pair of diseases: pneumonia and tuberculosis. Pneumonia, a disease that is accompanied by a high fever, among other things, is linked to a person's Luciferic tendency in a previous life. According to Steiner, the person had an inclination for the pleasures of the senses, particularly sex, in his previous life. In the world of the spirit, the need arises in the human being to compensate for the Luciferic influences, and he summons into his next life the circumstances that will enable him to come down with pneumonia. By overcoming the disease, the person acquires the forces necessary for subduing the Luciferic tendency. It should be mentioned that until about fifty years ago, recovery from pneumonia was not taken for granted. The big change that has taken place since then stems not only from the use of antibiotics, but also from the change in the nature of the disease, which is generally much less virulent than it was two generations ago.

The opposite disease is tuberculosis. Tuberculosis was very widespread throughout the world until about sixty or seventy years ago, when its incidence began to decrease, mainly in the developed countries. Tuberculosis is also a contagious disease that mainly attacks the lungs and progresses slowly for years. An immune reaction develops around the tuberculosis foci in the body, and a substance that isolates them sinks in and calcifies. This is a kind of self-healing attempt that actually works in many cases. Steiner links tuberculosis to a materialistic tendency in a past life, that is, to an Ahrimanic influence.

Tuberculosis is a chronic disease among whose

characteristics are long periods of a low-grade fever. This is in contrast to the high fever that erupts powerfully in the case of pneumonia. Tuberculosis is the colder and more prolonged of these two diseases, and it also causes calcification. It represents the diseases whose goal is to balance an Ahrimanic tendency. The feverish and turbulent pneumonia represents diseases that are meant to balance a Luciferic tendency.

It is important to stress that while the spiritual background of the disease is connected to the person's individual spiritual being, it stems from his previous incarnations in completely different living conditions. The examples presented here constitute a description of spiritual development, but under no circumstances do they constitute a moral judgment of the person who is sick with any kind of disease. After all, there is no one who isn't sick sometimes, just as there is no one who does not succumb to the two big tempters every now and then. Moreover, karma allows the disease to develop only in people who have acquired the strength that will enable them to grow through the disease. Other people, who do not yet have the requisite inner forces to overcome the disease, will continue to succumb to their Luciferic or Ahrimanic tendencies in their present lives as well.

Cancer and AIDS – modern diseases

Tuberculosis is a disease of an era. It is still common in various parts of the world, but it almost disappeared from developed countries in the middle of the twentieth century. At the same time, effective types of antibiotics against tuberculosis were discovered, but the disease had begun to wane even before the new medications had been introduced into broad use. While the conventional theory links the decrease in the incidence of the disease to a change in standard of living and in hygiene – and there is certainly more than a grain of truth in it – the high incidence of the disease also decreased in parts of the world where the living conditions had hardly changed at all. It has also been mentioned that at the same time, a change in the form and severity of pneumonia took place. Many other diseases appeared, changed beyond recognition, and also disappeared during the course of history, without any satisfactory explanation on the physical plane. The true reasons for changes in diseases are linked to the spiritual development of humanity. In recent generations, the Ahrimanic aberration has become more widespread and weighty than the Luciferic one, and the diseases through which karma helps the person overcome his weaknesses have also adapted themselves to the spirit of the times. Cancer has replaced tuberculosis as the disease that is typical of our times. The spiritual research of Rudolf Steiner links the various types of cancer to an Ahrimanic tendency. This is also true of many other diseases of our era, such as hypertension, heart diseases, diabetes and degenerative diseases of the nervous system. All of these diseases are meant to help the person overcome a defect of consciousness that is so common in the modern era: the perception of the world as a by-product of physical processes and of the human being as a creature without a past, a future or moral responsibility. In contrast to diseases such as cholera or pneumonia, which last for a limited amount of time and do not differ greatly from one person to the next, the modern illnesses are chronic and far more complex.

Cancer is a "cold" disease. Certain cells stop obeying the inner laws of the organism and produce a kind of foreign body, mass or lump in it, which is not a part of the human organism. Accelerated processes of calcification, destruction and loss of form take place in this lump, and these are characteristics of a disease that stems from an Ahrimanic aberration. At a later stage, pain and sometimes fever can occur, and they are actually more closely linked to a Luciferic disease. It has been mentioned that humankind strayed from the golden path of his development in the Ahrimanic direction after he had already fallen into Lucifer's net. In the individual, too, the Ahrimanic tendency is frequently added to a prior Luciferic tendency. This explains where the complexity of modern diseases such as cancer stems from. These diseases present the human being with a great challenge and at the same time enable him to overcome a large range of weaknesses that he is carrying in his soul from previous incarnations. Some two hundred different types of cancer exist, some common and some rare, some of which respond well to treatment and some of which do not. Even in cases of the same type of cancer, there are no two people who manifest the disease in an identical manner. Cancer is an individual disease to an extent that no disease before it has been. The person of today is more of an individual than in any previous time. Cancer, therefore, is linked at its spiritual basis to the present period in human development, just as the great epidemics were inextricably linked to human culture in other times[13].

Another modern disease, which demonstrates the principle of complexity in an obvious manner is the Acquired Immune Deficiency Syndrome, or AIDS. AIDS begins as a febrile illness and continues as a chronic and cold process of destruction of the immune system. As a result of the destruction of its immune capability, the organism is exposed to a long series of infectious diseases, some of them warm and some of them cold, as well as to various types of cancerous tumors. The individual differences between people who have AIDS are enormous. Some of them suffer damage to the digestive system, while others suffer damage to the nervous system, the respiratory system, or almost any other organ. This disease, which burst into human consciousness at the beginning of the 1980s, offers contemporary humanity the possibility of fortifying itself against a broad range of human weaknesses, whether Luciferic or Ahrimanic.

In our time, there has been a huge change in the sum total of possible diseases that people can contract. The achievements of modern medicine in the area of vaccinations against children's diseases, as well as the elimination of other contagious diseases, oblige karma to provide humanity with new diseases in order to ensure its continued development. AIDS is just the first of these diseases.

Another example is a disease that was rare and exotic until it suddenly took on a new form, which, in the last decade, has begun to pose a threat to the Western world. This disease is called Jakob-Kreuzfeld, a degenerative disease of the brain that is transmitted to human beings from the meat of infected animals. It is better known as "mad cow disease."

Let's go back to AIDS, which, as mentioned, burst into human consciousness at the beginning of the 1980s, immediately after the huge success of the World Health Organization in eliminating smallpox. At the end of the 1970s, the WHO completed a global immunization program that led to the elimination of the disease that had afflicted humankind for thousands of years. Like every other thing in our world, the constellation of circumstances described – the death of one disease and the birth of another – is not coincidental[14].

Congenital diseases

There are diseases that accompany the person his entire life. The physical basis for some of them is hereditary. The direct cause of such a disease is some kind of defect in the genetic makeup the fetus receives from his mother or father, or a defect that is the result of an unsuccessful combination of genes from both parents. There are many types of congenital diseases. Some of them are caused by a metabolic disorder, which is a disorder in the production or breakdown of one of the many substances that are essential for the building of the body and its normal growth. Other diseases can be expressed in a syndrome that is characterized by the typical appearance of all the children who suffer from it. The best known of the syndromes is Down's syndrome, which was the most common one until recent decades. Congenital diseases, both the metabolic disorders and the syndromes, can cause physical defects and defects in mental or intellectual functions.

People with congenital diseases often live lives that differ from what are considered normal lives in many realms. They require more help from the people close to them, not only during childhood, but sometimes for their whole lives. Some of them will not be able to lead independent lives at all and will need a supportive and helping community, a kind of substitute family, in adulthood. They are also liable to be limited in the professions they will practice, and some of them will be able to make their productive contribution to the world only in protective frameworks that are not exposed to real economic competition.

However, these people also make a crucial contribution to society in general and to those close to them in particular. In a society that contains such powerful egoistic forces, a society that operates according to Darwinian principles and in which the strong trample the weak underfoot – especially in the economic realm – disadvantaged people enable the "normal" person to overcome his egoism and work on behalf of the Other. They open a door to the whole of humanity and enable the forces of spiritual kindness to flow into earthly life. The highest manifestation of love is working for other people without expecting any reward. The people whose very existence depends on the good will of others bestow the gift of love on humanity.

In the last years of his life, Rudolf Steiner, who died in 1925, managed to lay the foundations of a broad movement of curative education that provided a framework of study, work and living for thousands of children and adults with special needs. Whenever Steiner spoke about karma, he made sure not to make generalizations or develop theories, but rather to describe concrete cases of people, alive or dead. This was also the case when he spoke about reasons that cause people to choose to incarnate with a disability. Some of these reasons will be mentioned briefly below in order to demonstrate the large range of situations that lead a human being to making such a choice.

One example is of people who, in their previous lives, were condemned to suffer sensory deprivation for one reason or another. They may have voluntarily chosen to eschew any experience of the physical world around them, or may have been prevented by other people from having such an experience during their lives. As a result, when they were in the spiritual world prior to being reborn, they did not have the knowledge of the physical world that is necessary for incarnating properly. Their spiritual being did not know how to build a physical body or how to enter it. These human beings choose future parents who will transmit defective organs to them via heredity[15].

Somewhere else, Steiner described three consecutive incarnations of a particular human being[16]. In the first life, the person's soul displayed superficiality and capriciousness, and refrained from devoting itself to anyone or anything. In the next life, after a sojourn in the spiritual world, these mental traits caused a more serious defect that expressed itself in a moral flaw this time – the tendency to lie. This does not refer to small, conventional lies, but real deception. In the world of the soul at the end of his second incarnation, this human being experienced the most powerful self-rejection. As a result, he made sure to seek flawed organs for himself in order to attain a life of difficulty that would afford him the self healing he yearned for.

People who experienced torture or a violent death in their previous lives will also have a hard time creating a normal life body and physical body for themselves when they are approaching their next life on earth. Another situation in which a human being can choose to be born with a disability involves people who have reached a high level of spiritual development. When they shape their next lives, these people might choose to incarnate in bodies that will cause them to lead a life of adversity. They do this so that by means of the difficulty, they can develop properties they identify as necessary for the continuation of their development.

Nowadays, however, rebirth is becoming more and more difficult for many of the human beings who choose to be born with disabilities. In all of the Western countries, the public health services fund a whole series of tests for pregnant women. The aim is to identify any suspected birth defect in the fetus right in the early stages of pregnancy. If a defect that is physical and localized is discovered – for example, a hole in the wall that divides the ventricles in the heart – most gynecologists and pregnant women opt to continue the pregnancy. If a disorder that is not limited to a particular organ, or which has implications for the mental or intellectual aspects, is suspected, the prevailing practice is to terminate the pregnancy by an abortion. Souls in need of a life with disabilities can almost no longer be born in a normal birth to an average family in developed countries. Souls that began an incarnation process in a fetus and experienced the traumatic termination of the pregnancy will seek other ways of being born as quickly as possible.

While advanced medical technology has blocked many possibilities of life with a disability from birth, it has also created new ones. Pregnancies that used to end with the death of the fetus because of a maternal medical problem or a premature birth culminate in the birth of a live infant today. Newborns with a birth weight of a few hundred grams can survive today thanks to the revolutionary advances in the care of premature infants. Despite the sophisticated and devoted care, in some cases these infants suffer damage during the problematic pregnancy, during the birth, or even as a result of the medical treatment. They carry this damage with them all their lives in many forms, cerebral palsy for instance. Cerebral palsy is the name given to brain damage that results in a disability in movement and speech. Sometimes – certainly not always – there is also damage to mental or intellectual abilities. This is one way in which human beings who need a life of disability from birth manage to bypass the barrier of abortion.

The last decades of the twentieth century witnessed a rise of hundreds of percent in the number of children with autistic traits diagnosed in the developed countries. While no flaws are identified in these children at birth, a problem of communication with their surroundings is discovered during early childhood, in addition to other mental problems. There have been attempts to link the unexplained rise in the number of afflicted children to various factors, among them the measles vaccination, which was introduced precisely during those years. This theory caused broad repercussions in the media, but did not receive the support of the doctors and scientists who hastened to check it out[17]. Two phenomena that occur at the same time can both reflect a higher truth without necessarily being linked to each other in a cause-and-effect relationship.

While researchers may succeed in finding a statistical link between the rise in the incidence of autism and various phenomena in the physical world, the real reason for the great increase in incidence will only be revealed to the eyes of the spiritual researcher. A change that operates so deeply inside human destiny stems from the aspiration of the spiritual hierarchies to help human beings who are on their way to be reborn to realize their karma. Are these human beings that choose to be born with autistic traits the ones that were previously denied their original choice of incarnation by external intervention?

Accidents and disasters

Although they are not diseases, accidents, natural disasters and man-made disasters also belong to the discussion. After all, they can also end in a life of disability, and it is difficult to distinguish between disabilities caused by them and disabilities caused by various diseases. People who suffer head injuries in road accidents, wars, terrorist attacks or other circumstances at a young age suffer from similar problems to those of people who were afflicted with cerebral palsy at birth. Thus, in a discussion about the link between diseases and destiny, it is appropriate to pay attention to the events that come from the outside and play a crucial part in people's lives.

From the point of view of Western medicine, not only accidents and disasters come from the outside, but also the various diseases that afflict people. This is the conventional way of thinking with regard to diseases that are caused by pathogens such as bacteria and viruses. However, other diseases such as cardiac and vascular diseases are greatly influenced by external factors: a diet rich in fats, smoking, and other risk factors. When the point of view stems from the subjective mental experience of the person, everything that is linked to the physical world becomes external. Even the person's genetic makeup – the location where the magic key that will close the Pandora's box of diseases is being sought today – is something external. People who are ill with serious diseases are provided with explanations regarding their disease by physicians. These explanations include up-to-date and reliable medical information. However, as has already been mentioned, no genetic, biochemical or microbiological truth supplies the answer to the question the sick person asks himself: Why me? Anthroposophy's answer to that basic question stems from its view of the person as a developing spiritual being. In order to fortify himself and overcome his weaknesses, the human being, during the interval between death and a new birth, chooses the situations by means of which he will be able to grow in the next incarnation on earth. From the spiritual point of view, no disease – and in most cases no accident either – lands on the person from the outside.

The person's everyday consciousness is completely unaware of the way in which the karma operates. Earlier on, we described how the human "I" returns to the spiritual world every night and is nourished once again by the higher spiritual consciousness that belonged to it in the life before birth. From the same higher spiritual consciousness, the impulses that motivate the person to meet his karma flow directly to the unconscious sphere of the soul – to the will. The person thinks he knows why he chances upon certain places and circumstances, but generally his reasons belong to the external surface. Only infrequently is the person likely to feel a vague, albeit very powerful, feeling that something momentous is about to happen. In any event, the ones who do know are the legs that carry the person toward his destiny. A person reaches some place in order to be exposed to germs that cause a certain disease. A person reaches another place in order to be exposed to an accident that belongs to his karma no less than the germs do. In the same way that the person's genetic makeup exposes him to the possibility of succumbing to various diseases that will only be realized as a result of his habits and mental traits, so the potential for accidents that is buried deep in the unconscious layers of his soul will only be realized if the soul and spiritual conditions for it are created.

Is what is true for individual events, such as diseases or accidents, also valid for events that involve the fate of groups of people? In the past, people were more vulnerable to natural disasters. Epidemics decimated the populations of entire continents. Even if the victims of earthquakes and floods were initially rescued, they later succumbed to disease and starvation. Today, human beings know how to diminish the suffering engendered by natural disasters, but they have made sure that there is a substitute for them in the form of man-made disasters. Road accidents are one of the modern substitutes – modest but effective – for natural disasters. Leaks from chemical plants or nuclear reactors are also substitutes – less modest ones.

In the face of a disaster involving many people, we can ask whether in fact the individual karma of each of them led them to the unavoidable disaster. Rudolf Steiner's response to this question was negative[16]. Among the hundreds or thousands of casualties in an earthquake, for instance, there will also be many whose karma did not request the earthquake. However, in the world of the spirit, no human experience is lost or "wasted". When people are exposed to a particular disaster that is not linked to the karma they are carrying from the past, the disaster still becomes the driving force of their future karma. If a person survives some kind of disaster, the experience becomes an influence that is at work in him for the rest of his life. This influence will keep on exerting itself on his life in the worlds of the soul and spirit and will contribute to his next life. If the person dies in the disaster, the circumstances of his death will certainly accompany him for the entire duration of his journey in the spiritual world and will play a central role in shaping his next life on earth.

Even if a certain disaster is in no way linked to the karma of a particular person, it is certainly linked to the karma of the group to which that person belongs. When a person receives into his individual destiny something that belongs to the destiny of a human community, he contributes to the spiritual progress of the entire community. A soldier who dies in battle assumes something of the karma of the nation or country for which he sacrificed his life. A person who dies in an epidemic assumes a part of the karma of the era in which he lives, and it would not be incorrect to identify the element of sacrifice in his disease and in his death as well. Nowadays, these things are valid, for instance, with regard to people that suffer from the "epidemics" of the New Age. No one who struggles with a disease such as cancer or AIDS strengthens only his own spiritual "I", but rather contributes in parallel to the spiritual development of the entire human community.

Healing

Illness as a healing force

It is difficult to describe a greater discrepancy between two points of view, than the one that exists between the regular perception of disease and the spiritual one. By their very nature, spiritual truths – including those that deal with illness and healing – frequently differ from any conventional thought or belief. Overall, the discussion of spiritual questions demands a lot more from the reader than ordinary reading. First and foremost, he has to display a great deal of openness. A person who already knows everything about life cannot learn anything new. He has to liberate himself, at least temporarily, from his old views and opinions in order to accord his thinking the requisite space and time for examining new ideas. Second, he also has to be able to put some emotional distance between himself and the questions under discussion. When the person himself or someone in his immediate surroundings is afflicted with a disease, a discussion of this kind undoubtedly arouses strong emotions in him. He will have to put aside not only old opinions, but also the emotions that are evoked in him, and that is even more difficult. And finally, the person is, of course, also required to invest forces of will and thinking. Spiritual truths cannot be grasped by someone who reads someone else's words quietly and passively. Only someone who makes an effort to think can really discover the significance and the value of the words.

It has already been said that the human being chooses the disease out of spiritual consciousness while he is between death and a new birth in the spiritual world. The disease is meant to help him overcome weaknesses that were expressed in his previous life. The previous chapter described the human being's two major deviations from the path of development that the higher beings of the spiritual world mapped out for him. One is the egoistic deviation, which motivates many of his deeds, among them deeds that are perceived as bad, but also deeds that are perceived as positive – a work of art, for instance. The spiritual being that tempted the human being to free himself from the protection of the gods and gave him the experience of a sense of self and the attendant egoism is the being that was revealed to Adam and Eve in the form of a snake – Lucifer in the modern mythology of Anthroposophy. The human being's second deviation is the blindness to the spiritual source of things and the perception of the world as a random physical occurrence that has neither direction nor purpose. The spiritual power that charted the course of human development to the point of almost forgetting the spiritual world and clinging to material things is called Ahriman. How exactly does illness enable the person to find his spiritual path between these two spiritual influences?

The spiritual being of the person overcomes the Luciferic temptation through pain. Pain accompanies the "warm" diseases, which are patently Luciferic diseases.

However, pain is also present in the "cold" diseases. Cancer, for instance, is a "cold" disease that causes some people to suffer severe pain. The same is true for some diseases of the joints, which are diseases of cold and calcification that affect elderly people. This stems from the fact that every person of our time bears in his karma both the Luciferic temptation and the Ahrimanic error, which have accumulated during the course of many incarnations. The "modern" illnesses stem from this complex karma, and so they are also more complex than the diseases of the past.

During the expulsion from Eden, Eve is told that she would give birth in sorrow. The moment of birth in the woman's life is the moment in which she is compelled to give up, at least partially, her sense of self and accept another human being into her soul. From this moment on, she is supposed to worry about the infant's needs first of all, and only then her own. The pains that accompany the birth are connected to her relinquishing of her sense of self, which is a triumph over the Luciferic being[18]. Any situation in which the person's soul opens up to receive and love another person, and not in order to gain any kind of reward, is a triumph of that kind.

Pain is caused when the person's soul body, in reaction to a stimulus or to a process of a disease, penetrates and takes hold of a particular organ too tightly. The normal situation in which the higher bodies enter the lower ones is when the person awakes from sleep. The excessive penetration of the soul body into the life body and the physical body is a kind of local process of awakening that is exceptional in its intensity. The normal presence of the soul body in the organ is sufficient for its everyday functioning, but does not contain an awareness of the organ itself. The soul body penetrates the person's hand to the required extent in order to move it. If the soul body penetrates the hand too strongly because of a bruise or an inflammation, the person suddenly becomes aware of its presence. This is the feeling of pain. Just as a child puts his hand in the fire and the pain teaches him not to do it again, so it is with the human being. He experiences the pain that accompanies the disease. The pain is the expression in the present life of the fierce desire for self healing that he experienced in the spiritual world prior to birth. In this sense, which is so different from the person's earthly experience, the pain is a healing force.

The disease enables the person to cope with the Ahrimanic error as well. The force that overcomes Ahriman is the force that is born in the spiritual being of the person as a result of the physical destruction and the loss of function that occur in the diseased organs. Untreated tuberculosis destroys the lungs in a process most of whose stages do not cause pain. The chronic forms of viral hepatitis, hepatitis B and C, are liable to bring about the slow destruction of the liver, which is not accompanied by pain. Most types of cancer often reach a very advanced stage without causing pain. The above mentioned diseases – and others as well – that cause the destruction of an organ and the loss of its function, serve the person's higher spiritual consciousness that aspires to cleanse itself of the erroneous illusion from its previous life. Following the destruction of the organs of the physical body, the human being is aroused to a spiritual recognition that his own existence is separate from the existence of the physical organs, and is not dependent on them. Once again, he discovers his true home that is hidden behind the physical – the world of the spirit.

What has been said up till now must evoke serious questions in every reader, however open to new ideas he may be. For instance, a question concerning pain: In the light of the spiritual significance that is attributed to pain, is the use of painkillers justified? And another question that borders on the absurd but must nonetheless be asked: Is it right to fight a disease and prevent it from destroying the organs of the body when we are aware of the importance of the destruction?

The unequivocal answer is that from the spiritual point of view, there is no substitute for fighting the disease. The sick person, with the forces of his everyday consciousness, fights the disease by overcoming fear, selfishness, pride and hopelessness. Coping with the disease – relentless coping, sometimes against all odds – develops forces of courage and love in the person's soul. Courage is acquired through the struggle with fear. Love is the fruit of the person's becoming resigned to his life. It is the force by means of which he forgives himself and accepts his weaknesses and his disease. It is the force that is the opposite of egoism and empty pride. Receiving treatment for lowering the level of pain or for halting the destruction process caused by the disease is part of the person's way of coping. When a person makes use of his disease in order to conquer fear and egoism, every treatment he receives for his disease or pain contributes to the growth of the healing forces in his soul.

So much for the person himself. Medical personnel also have to fight the disease with every available means. A physician who weighs up whether or not to apply a certain treatment to a person out of considerations that ostensibly relate to that person's karma, is acting out of arrogance and is himself in danger of falling into Lucifer's net. The concern with the karma should be left to the beings of love and grace that are responsible for it, and the physician must do everything possible to heal the person.

Nevertheless, the treatment of the sick person must be based on common sense. Treatment with the most advanced medical technologies does not always serve the good of the patient. Sometimes, a powerful technology that is employed without due consideration will cause more harm than good. Painkillers must also be used judiciously. Before his death, the cancer patient must receive treatment against pain, if he is suffering from pain. However, high dosages of painkillers will cause him not to be lucid, so that he will not be able to take leave of his dear ones when he is fully alert. He is also liable to die before he has finished setting his affairs in order and is ready to die in peace, since painkillers affect the respiratory center in the brain and suppress the sick person's breathing. When treating pain, the objective must be to moderate the person's suffering so that he will not curse the day he was born, but also to maintain as much as possible his lucid state of soul, so he will be able to make the best use of this very special and decisive time in his life.

Consciousness and healing

In certain situations, human consciousness can have a healing effect on the person's soul body and life body. First, the person can sometimes prevent disease by the power of his consciousness. Rudolf Steiner describes a person who, while he was not actually an egoist, lived his life in complete self-involvement and did not take an interest in the world around him[16]. After residing in the spiritual world, the same human being was born to his new life with two karmic consequences in his possession. The first was a tendency toward delusion and self-deception that stemmed directly from his lack of interest in the world in his previous life. The second was the need to contract measles, which could compensate for the weakness. These two tendencies, one mental and the other physical, are the two facets of one spiritual essence. Steiner, who spoke about the karma of the person from direct spiritual experience, relates that the person succeeded in fortifying his soul so that it no longer tended toward delusion and deceit, and in that way canceled out his karma's need for measles. The case described above was rare, apparently, even when measles was still a common disease. Many souls requested self healing by means of measles, since the mental weakness of a lack of interest in the world was widespread during certain periods. However, most of them preferred to go through the strengthening experience of the disease at a young age and avoid the need to fight a life of self-deception by means of their consciousness.

A person can develop self-knowledge, heal his soul from innate weaknesses and thus prevent a disease that is supposed to occur later in life. Is it possible to cure an existing disease with the power of consciousness as well? Yes, it is possible to affect and sometimes even cure diseases intentionally so long as they have not yet penetrated the physical body. Such an influence begins with the activity of the "I". The person presents certain pictures to his soul and focuses his entire attention on them. This spiritual and soul activity must be repeated every day at a regular time for at least a few minutes. The picture that he presents to his soul can be a picture of sunlight penetrating his body via his senses, flowing through his head and gradually filling his entire body, from his chest to his abdomen and limbs. When the person nurtures images like these in his soul, they affect his soul body first and foremost, and this in turn affects his life body. The connection of the soul body to the life body is the birthplace of the diseases that are considered psychosomatic. By creating a regular rhythm of nourishing the soul with such an image, it is even possible to cure diseases of this kind, diseases that have not yet taken hold of the physical body[19]. Besides the image of sunlight filling the body, there are other images that serve the same purpose. By means of the image, the person opens himself up to the influence of the spiritual beings that accompany humankind and the karma of every individual. The physical sunlight is what makes life on earth possible. It is the pictorial image of the forces of love and grace that flow from these "sun beings" all the time and are the spiritual source of our lives here on earth.

In this way, the person can act on himself with the power of consciousness in a way that can sometimes, but not always, lead to complete healing. When more serious diseases are involved, the person can still help himself to a certain extent by means of his consciousness, but he will also need medical treatment that works where the consciousness cannot penetrate. In every chronic disease that involves the physical body, there is a pattern of improvement and deterioration. The deterioration that recurs after an improvement has been achieved stems from instability in the relationship between the life body and the physical body. The cause of this instability is the negative influence of the soul body on the life body. When the person's soul is constantly full of thoughts and images of illness and pain, it exerts an influence that is opposite to the one that was described in the process of self-healing. The image of light and grace, when it lives in the soul, can affect the soul body and the life body and lead to healing. The incessant preoccupation with pain and suffering also spills over from the soul and affects the life body via the soul body – not in a positive way, but rather in a manner that increases the above mentioned instability[16].

In such a situation, the person can use the power of consciousness to try to clear his soul of the constant preoccupation with the disease. It is important to mention that it is a matter of a completely different mental activity from the denial of the disease or the suppression of its seriousness – two psychological defense mechanisms often used by sick people. While he is completely conscious of his disease and its seriousness, the person chooses to distance the disease-related contents from his soul in order to make room for healthy contents. He can do this, for instance, if he occupies himself with helping others. He can also draw forces from observing natural processes such as blooming and flowering or the setting sun – preferably at regular times. The difficulty is to make sure to fill his soul with the new content without allowing the old content to sneak back in. Another activity that can serve the same purpose is the study of spiritual material. When a person fills his soul with questions and ideas from the spiritual realm, his threshold of tolerance for the pains and the distress increases. The influence of the conscious activity on the disease in this case is not direct, but it can be very significant.

Many people who suffer from chronic or disabling diseases live their lives intensely and do not allow the disease to rear its head and control them. Most of them reached this way of coping with their ailment by themselves, without reading or hearing about it from someone else. Through their perpetual struggle against hardships, they acquire the power to overcome the weaknesses that reside in their karma. However, anyone who knows such people also receives a bit of healing for his soul from them via the daily testimony to the valor of the spirit and its victory over the limitations of the body.

Psychic healing

Sometimes one person can transmit healing forces to another. The process is similar to that of self-healing, which occurs by means of reinforcing the forces of the soul by immersing oneself in the image of sunlight. When it occurs between two people, it begins in the soul body of the one who is stronger than normal as a result of processes that he is usually unaware of. The soul body of the "healer" transmits his strength to his life body, and from there the healing effect flows to the life body of the sick person. The occurrence of "spiritual healing", "psychic healing" or "magnetic healing", to mention just three of the names that are used to describe this phenomenon, depends on the fact that the "healer" feels fierce compassion for the patient. The source of this compassion lies in the special karmic connection that exists between them, even though it is highly likely that they do not know each other in their present lives. As in the case of self-healing, the effect is not strong enough for healing the physical body, but rather for healing the disease processes that are located in the soul body or the life body. Since we are talking about a phenomenon that stems from a karmic connection between two individuals, and since the presence of healing forces in the soul body of the "healer" is instinctive and not the fruit of conscious spiritual training, after the original role of the healing forces ends, they become weaker. When the "healer" turns his exceptional talents into an occupation, there is not a lot of them left, in most cases. What began as a flow of healing force between two individuals is liable to end up in disappointment for other people who are seeking salvation from their sufferings and end up disillusioned[19].

Things were not like that in the past. In past eras, the human being had not yet distanced himself so much from the direct experience of the spiritual world. The connection between his soul and spirit being and his life body was tighter because his life body was not yet rooted so firmly in his physical body as it is today. In other words, spiritual and soul influences operated with far greater intensity on the life body. The life body, in turn, because of its relative freedom from the physical body, was able to exert a healing influence on it from the outside. In the Judeo-Christian traditions, many miraculous acts of healing are described. Elijah, Elisha and Isaiah healed by means of spiritual powers, but were also assisted by physical means such as warmth or dried figs. The exceptional healing deeds of Christ are widely described in the New Testament. The Gospel of Luke, who himself was a physician, stresses the archetypal nature of these acts of healing. Indeed, it is possible to learn from the Gospel about the healing effects that flowed from the spiritual "I" of Christ to the various bodies of the people who turned to him for salvation. Among these acts of healing were the healing of those possessed by demons, relating to the soul body; the restoration of movement to a lame man, which is apparently the healing of the life body; and the healing of a leper and of a woman who had been bleeding for twelve years, which are acts of healing that work all the way through to the physical body[20].

That was the case some two thousand years ago. We also know from other ancient cultures, in both East and West, that sick people would turn to the priest in the temple. The priest used spiritual healing forces as well as such means as herbal remedies or even surgery. Humanity has come a long way since then. The vivid consciousness of the physical world dominates human life today. The spiritual world has been forgotten, and it constitutes a vague memory that is preserved in ancient books and folk legends. The life body is closer to the physical body and to the influences it absorbs through it from the physical surroundings. The effect of the person's spiritual and soul being on the lower bodies is weaker than ever today. However, human evolution is still far from complete. The human being has distanced himself from the spiritual world as a result of the Luciferic temptation, and has been bound tightly to the physical world by means of the Ahrimanic influence. He has distanced himself from the guidance of the gods and has gained a sense of self. The period in which we live is a period in which the person himself manages the world around him, for better or for worse. Like an adolescent who develops his power of judgment through countless mistakes, so humanity in its entirety navigates its steps along its path to the future, when it will join up with the spiritual world once more. The human being who finds his way back to the gods will not be an ignorant creature as in the past, but rather a spiritual being that has achieved independence and can work together with the hierarchies of the spiritual world. Already in the next few millennia – a short time in cosmic terms – the human being will once more develop the conscious connection to the spiritual world. In parallel, a certain distance between the life body and the physical body will gradually develop, and this will once again permit the flow of the healing influences from one person to another.

The signs that herald what is hidden in the future are the first self-healing abilities that people are attaining right now by the power of their consciousness. In contrast, in the spontaneous phenomena of transferring healing forces from one person to the other, it is possible to see remnants of the past. However, the reality of today is such that complete healing of serious and chronic diseases by means of the consciousness is not the province of humanity. Therefore, the correct way of coping with disease must address all of the four human bodies. It is necessary to work on the physical body by physical means. The life body must be nourished with life forces. And of course, it is necessary to relate to the person's soul and to his immortal spiritual being. The approach that is satisfied with the treatment of the physical body only is the Ahrimanic approach. The aspiration to turn to the higher being of the person only is the Luciferic aspiration. Following is the way to treat the whole human being.

Treating the whole human being

In order to treat the sick person, the physician uses medications. The medications act on the physical body and, through it, on the entire being of the person. The medications that are very widely used today in every country are the chemical medications that are manufactured in the giant plants of the global drug industry. Most of the chemical or "conventional" medications, as they are called, are very effective in the treatment of people who have certain diseases. Frequently they save lives or alleviate situations of extreme distress. Children with leukemia were virtually sentenced to death forty years ago. Today, the vast majority of children with various types of leukemia are cured thanks to the new medications that successfully attack and destroy the cancer cells. Infectious diseases that ended in death or serious disability half a century ago are treated successfully today with various new antibiotics. This is the case with bacterial meningitis, for instance.

In most cases, conventional medications only create a problem when they are used excessively. When a child who suffers from recurrent ear infections receives antibiotic treatment for weeks and months, bacteria that are resistant to the antibiotic might develop in his body, causing the ear infection to spread to nearby organs – the meninges, for instance. When a person who suffers from a type of cancer that does not respond to chemotherapy – this is only effective against certain types of cancer – receives treatment with these extremely powerful drugs anyway, the disease is not affected, but the immune system is. Since Western medicine does not have medications other than chemical ones, they are often administered needlessly. In many cases, in fact, the damage caused by the medications exceeds their benefit[21].

There are also medications that are not manufactured in factories but are produced from nature. These medications, which are taken from the mineral, plant and animal kingdom, are closer to humans in several ways. First, they belong to nature, that is, they belong to the whole of humanity and it is impossible to patent them and earn millions from them. Second, they are created in the great workshop of the Creator from the same spiritual sources from which the human bodies were formed. The person takes the source of the remedy, a plant for instance, and uses it without turning it into something that is alien to nature. The processes that plant remedies undergo include drying, simmering, distilling or dilution to tiny doses. These processes aim to extract the healing property from the raw material and preserve it or even reinforce it. In modern medicine, too, use is sometimes made of·

medications from plant sources, except that then, in general, the aim is to isolate one chemical component that has been identified as the active substance from the sum total of the hundreds of chemical substances present in the plant. In this kind of process, the character of the plant as a whole entity whose sum total of chemical components expresses its life body is lost. Among the medications produced from plants are various types of antibiotics as well as types of chemotherapy for cancer. These medications, which are generally extremely powerful and effective, unleash destructive forces that destroy the bacteria or the cancer cells. However, they lack the complementary and balancing properties of the whole plant, the properties that reinforce the healthy functioning of the organism. The one-sided action of the chemical medication is opposed to the healing nature of the plant, which is after all a spiritual entity that is inextricably connected to the spiritual evolution of humanity.

In spite of – or perhaps because of – the affinity between natural remedies and humans, the natural remedies are also liable to cause damage if carelessly used. Many plants can cause acute allergic reactions no less than chemical substances. Some of the most powerful known toxins are derived from plants or animals. Ancient spiritual knowledge enabled humankind to use these very toxins as powerful medications after they had been transformed by dilution or some other process. In ancient times, the knowledge that enabled plants and minerals to be utilized correctly after undergoing the appropriate preparation processes was the province of the priests in the temples and in the mystery centers. Via these places, the spiritual hierarchies bestowed their goodness on humanity, goodness that included the wisdom of healing. We have already described the course of human evolution, which caused spiritual wisdom and its sources to be gradually forgotten and abandoned. In general, even people who use natural remedies nowadays do not fully understand the mode of action of the various plants. In the future, the properties of the natural remedies will shift even further from the field of human knowledge, unless new spiritual research enables the contemporary person once more to attain spiritual knowledge of every plant and mineral. Then human consciousness will again be able to recognize the connection between the diseases of humanity and the healing forces of nature. However, until then, it is important to remember that sometimes there is no substitute for the chemical medications and innovative medical technologies that save lives in many situations. The use of chemical medications as well as of plant remedies must arise from knowledge of their properties and their limitations, and from an awareness of the sum total of their effects on the person's physical, soul and spiritual being[22].

Chemical medications work on the physical body and, through it, on the rest of the bodies. Natural remedies or treatments frequently work directly on the life body, the soul body or even the "I". For instance, homeopathic preparations, which are diluted many times until a separation between the physical substance and its inherent healing property is achieved, directly affect the life body. Ointments or compresses that contain the essence of some plant work externally on the skin and are initially absorbed by the person's senses. In other words, they directly affect the soul body in which all the sensory processes occur. In this case, too, only knowledge of the whole human being can afford an understanding of how the treatment works. Physical knowledge is incapable of explaining how an ointment, whose components are not absorbed through the skin at all, succeeds in working on internal organs.

By means of treatment, it is possible to affect the person's spiritual being, the "I", as well. Such an effect will be achieved, for instance, by hot or sometimes cold baths or compresses that raise or lower the temperature of the body or the organ. Through warmth the spiritual "I" takes hold of the physical body and the physical organs. By means of such a simple method, such as warming or cooling, it is possible to affect the intensity and the manner in which the person's spiritual being takes hold of his body.

External treatments such as baths, compresses or massages address the person's higher bodies through water, air and warmth. There are other methods that address the person's higher bodies, such as acquiring new behavior patterns. The immediate example of the link between a behavior pattern and health is the broad domain of nutrition. The accepted perception of nutrition is part of the natural sciences and therefore does not relate to nutrition as a bridge to the person's higher bodies. It hardly relates to the quality of the food, either. The main area nutritional science deals with is the chemical composition of the food: carbohydrates, fats, calories and so on. The reason for this is that modern science knows how to break down and count but does not have the faintest idea what quality is.

There is a large qualitative difference between vegetarian and meat nutrition, for instance. This goes beyond the differences in fat or protein content. Plant-based nutrition contains life forces but not soul forces. As a result, digestion requires a much greater presence of the human soul body than with meat nutrition. The undigested fiber, which constitutes a large part of the plant mass, forces the soul body and the human "I" to make an effort. The vigorous digestive action that results from fiber-rich nutrition can attest to the lively involvement of the soul body in the digestive system. In the long run, the cumulative effect of vegetarian nutrition on the person's soul is the development of strong will forces. In contrast, a meat meal, which contains elements of an animal soul body that is alien to the human organism, causes the higher bodies to distance themselves slightly from the digestive system. This phenomenon is expressed, for example, in the need to doze off after a meat meal. There are also circumstances in which meat nutrition is more suitable for the person's needs – for instance, during periods when he is under great pressure and stress. In these situations, the diminished presence of the higher bodies in the digestive system releases soul forces for the use of the person who is bearing the load.

Besides the type and amounts of food the person eats, it is also very important how and when he eats. Orderly eating at regular times is a prerequisite for the health of the life body. The person's life forces are no less affected by the rhythm of his life than by the food he eats. Every person who has succeeded in losing weight by means of a nutritional change knows that orderly, moderate eating at regular times is no less important for maintaining the weight level than the amount of calories in the food. Why moderate? When the person sits down to eat, he must not only sit his physical body down, but also his soul. If his soul continues to race, clinch deals and make plans during the meal, it occupies a relatively large volume of the soul body and prevents it from dedicating itself more to the act of digestion. In less modern societies, people knew this secret and would say a blessing or offer thanks, before and after the meal. This served as a kind of pause that summons the person's spiritual "I" to take hold of the reins of the soul body, at least for a short time.

Conventional nutritional science, which relates only to the physical components of food and to the person's physical body, is repeatedly being shown to be incompatible with reality. The outstanding historical example is what was preached to women for decades during the twentieth century: not to breast-feed their infants, but rather to give them milk substitutes that had been formulated according to the most advanced scientific knowledge of those days. Even today, when the marvelous and inimitable uniqueness of mother's milk is no longer in dispute, the blindness of the experts resonates in the advertisements for sophisticated milk substitutes, most of which are – not surprisingly – manufactured by the same giant companies of global industry.

Another example from the 1970s and 80s was how the medical establishment mobilized to encourage the sale of margarine, following the discovery of the link between high cholesterol levels and cardiac and vascular diseases. Margarine is vegetable fat that has undergone industrial processing in order to rid it completely of its life forces. As a vegetable product, it does not contain the cholesterol that is produced only by animals. As a dead substance, however, it creates a heavy burden on the human liver and causes the liver itself to produce excessive levels of cholesterol. Today, the nutrition experts also know that even though margarine does not contain cholesterol, it raises the cholesterol levels, while cold-pressed olive oil, which preserves its life forces, lowers cholesterol levels through its beneficial effect on the liver. Today, too, nutritional recommendations that people are given by the medical system still do not relate to the most important subject, which is the quality of the food[23].

Many books have been and will be written about nutrition. By virtue of its being a central component in the contemporary perception of health, we have briefly discussed nutrition in order to stress three points. The first point is the tremendous limitation of the materialistic scientific theory when it aspires to operate in real life. The second point is the healing ability inherent in the understanding of nutrition that is based on knowledge of the whole person. The third point presents nutrition as an example of an accumulation of habits, which affect the person's health. Habits in other domains such as physical activity, hygiene, emotional reaction, and even thinking patterns, are also closely connected to the person's health. The earlier the correct habits are instilled, the deeper their effect is for the human being.

In contrast to nutrition, the next domain is not perceived by most people as exerting a direct effect on health and illness. We are referring to art. Art therapy affects not only the soul but also the body, with every therapy having its own mode of action. Three of the therapies that are used in anthroposophic medicine will be presented here as examples. The first is curative eurythmy. It is a method of movement which works directly on the life body. When a person speaks, each sound is produced by a different movement of the chest muscles, the vocal cords, the tongue, the palate and the lips. All these movements within the organism manifest externally as speech. The eurythmic movements are an outward expression of these internal movements. However, when the person performs these movements with his limbs, they exert a powerful effect in the opposite direction, that is, on his internal organs and his life forces. Each movement has its own quality, and by means of different movements, it is possible to create very specific formative effects on the life body, thus making eurythmy into a powerful therapy. When working with eurythmy for a long time, its effect can penetrate the physical body as well. This can be seen clearly in children, in whom the physical body is not yet hardened and is therefore more accessible to the healing effects.

Another therapy is painting or color therapy. One of the main techniques of color therapy involves applying water colors to slightly wet paper. The water element enables the paint to free itself of its mineral property and open up to absorb the movements of the person's soul, which are then expressed on the sheet of paper. By choosing and applying certain colors, an effect can be achieved that works from the sheet of paper through the person's eye and is absorbed in his soul. Since every color has its own special quality, it is possible to attain an intentional influence on the soul by means of the different colors and forms. Beyond their mental effect, colors also act on the bodies. Colors are expressions of light. The combination of all the colors of the rainbow creates the light that shines in the air. Therefore, colors mainly affect the soul body that is connected to the air element, and through it the life body, which serves as a kind of sound-box for the qualities that spread through the soul body.

The last example is speech therapy. Speech is one of the most pronounced expressions of the person's soul and spirit. A person who thinks clearly speaks differently from a person whose thoughts are confused. A calm person speaks differently from a stressed person. By means of certain speech exercises, the human "I" learns how it can strengthen its presence in the soul body. There are other art therapies, no less important, such as sculpture therapy or music therapy. We have presented three specific examples here in order to demonstrate the possibility of achieving specific effects on the bodies via the soul. Curative eurythmy works on the relationship between the life body and the physical body, color therapy works on the relationship between the soul body and the life body, and speech therapy works on the relationship between the "I" and the soul body. There are many treatment methods in the fields of complementary medicine that declare themselves to be "holistic" methods that address the whole person. However, if a method or therapy does not arise from true spiritual knowledge of the whole person – knowledge that goes into the small details of the mode of action of the person's spirit in his soul and body – then it is legitimate to question its holism.

Medications use the gate of the physical body in order to enter and act in the human being. Habits, food and external treatments mainly enter via the gate of the life body. The art therapies open the gate of the soul. And there is also a direct path to the human "I". The person can gain some understanding of his own spiritual being if he observes attentively its visible expression, which is his biography.

In the person's biography, two elements are joined: the general human one, and the individual one. Human development from childhood and youth to adulthood and old age first obeys general spiritual principles. An investigation of the biography identifies these general principles through the physical and mental processes that occur in most people of similar ages. The age when the milk teeth are replaced by the permanent teeth, for instance, teaches us about a new stage in the relationship between the physical body and the life body. The teeth are the first body parts that cease being filled with life forces and stop renewing themselves. The life forces that are being released gradually direct themselves toward the development of the child's thinking ability. During the stage of puberty, as well, forces are released – this time of the soul body. These forces are released particularly from the sex organs, but also from all the rest of the body's organs – the vocal cords for example – that go through a process of transformation at this age. Now the possibility of gradually starting to develop powers of judgment and of differentiation between right and wrong emerges in the young soul. Those are two examples of stages of bodily, soul and spiritual development that continues throughout the person's life[24]. Every human being pours the individual components of his karma into this general human mold. Thus the life of one person becomes completely different from the life of the next. The first brings with him an impressive thinking ability while the second brings powerful will forces. During their lives, they will have a few or many encounters and experiences, all in accordance with their individual karma.

When a person looks at his life systematically, he is likely to discover the common thread that passes through the various periods and ups and downs, and gives them meaning. When the inner connection between the events of his life becomes clear, he also begins to see the disease in a new light. First it was an alien thing that landed on him from the outside, and now he identifies it as a part of his life[25].

Looking at the biography creates an opening for the person to make peace in his soul with even the most painful events he has experienced. He will sometimes be able to forgive someone who hurt him and at the same time forgive himself as well. It has already been said that the human consciousness in our time is too weak to work directly on diseases that have taken hold of the physical body. The journey along the paths of the biography does not promise physical healing, but it can certainly lead to the healing of the wounds of the soul.

When does healing occur?

As we have already mentioned, healing can be related to from various and even opposite directions. From the spiritual point of view, the disease is a process that enables the person to overcome weaknesses that he is carrying from previous lives. The person is cured of the Luciferic and

Ahrimanic deviations by means of experiencing pain and the loss of the function of body organs. For most contemporary people, those are theoretical notions that are completely detached from the aspiration to heal oneself that fills the consciousness of a person who has a serious disease. Cure, from the everyday point of view, is the restoration of normal functioning to the organs and the disappearance of pain. People who are suffering from a serious disease simply want to get up one morning and find that the disease is no longer there, that it has disappeared like a bad dream. Some of them – those who can see the disease as a part of their lives and seek to know what the lesson that it has come to teach them is – will indeed aspire to change their life in accordance with the new insights that the disease has given them. Ultimately, however, their main desire is to be healthy once more and get on with living their life.

The question to be asked is: What is the relationship between what is described as healing in its spiritual sense and healing in its everyday sense? Is healing in the spiritual sense always accompanied by "physical" healing? And the opposite question: Does "physical" healing necessarily indicate that the healing of the person's soul and spirit being has been achieved? The answer to neither question is self-evident.

We can try to answer these questions by means of anthroposophic spiritual knowledge, so long as we do not ask them about a specific person. When the question is asked about the destiny of an individual who is now fighting a disease, it is actually impossible to answer it because at least a part of the answer is still hidden in the future. Any attempt to extrapolate from the general spiritual laws to the destiny of a specific person is wrong at best and charlatan at worst. Only a person with direct spiritual vision could learn – if the spiritual world permits – what another person's destiny holds in store for him. However, a person who really sees spiritually will be extremely careful of jeopardizing the other person's spiritual freedom with spurious statements about his future. On the other hand, if the sick person himself devotes time and mental forces to studying spiritual thoughts, he will gradually recognize their importance for his own life. He may not have the privilege of seeing his future spread out before him – this is the picture that is revealed to the human being in the world of the spirit prior to birth – but he is definitely entitled to expect that the past will become clear to his gaze, that his life will reveal its hidden meaning to him.

So when does "physical" healing occur? A person who is sick with a disease and, through his suffering, overcomes the residual weaknesses from his previous lives, can continue living if the conditions of his surroundings enable him to make use of the new soul and spiritual forces he has acquired through his disease. The person's physical condition, the proper functioning of his internal organs, is perhaps the most important factor for the continuation of life. If as a result of the disease his body organs have been badly damaged, it is obvious that it will be difficult for him to keep on living, even if he has attained new soul forces. The person's higher being will aspire to return to the spiritual world in order to shape his next life on earth so that his new soul forces will be expressed in it. Other circumstances can also cause the human "I" to forgo the continuation of his life in the physical body. For instance, a person lives in a social, family or status setting that prevents him from giving the people around him what his soul could have given as a result of its new forces. This person's being will also aspire to the world of the spirit in order to shape the course of his next life there, so that his forces will be fully expressed and he will be able to give of them to the people with whom he is bound by destiny[16].

Up till now, the situation in which the person achieved the soul and spiritual development his higher being aspired to has been described, but this development is not necessarily accompanied by a healing process of the life body and the physical body. What about a person who does recover from his disease? Did he overcome the weaknesses of his soul? Did he accomplish the objectives of his karma?

Breast cancer is one of the most common diseases of our time. Its incidence is constantly rising in developed society and it is also occurring in younger women than in the past. If the cancer is detected early thanks to the alertness of the woman or the physician, it is often possible to cure it. When a lump that is suspected to be malignant is discovered in the breast, the woman undergoes surgery to remove it, and it is examined in order to see whether it in fact contains cancerous cells. If it is indeed malignant, it is often necessary to extend the surgery and extract the lymph nodes from the armpit region, since they drain the lymph from the breast and are liable to be infected. Sometimes the entire breast has to be removed, depending on the type of cancerous cells and their distribution. After the surgery, the physicians recommend that the woman undergo chemotherapy, which is spread over half a year and has some side effects. Most of the side effects are extremely unpleasant – for instance, hair loss or acute weakness and fatigue. A few of them are even liable to be dangerous. The next stage in the treatment is radiation, which is administered to the part of the breast that was not removed, and it also has side effects. The last stage is frequently hormonal treatment that must be taken for several years – generally in the form of oral tablets. The procedure described is one of a range of possibilities. In each woman with breast cancer, the treatment may vary according to her condition. However, every woman who has breast cancer and undergoes this treatment in part or in its entirety concomitantly goes through difficult trials of fear and suffering. Through the experience of suffering, she copes with the Luciferic temptation, and by overcoming her fear, she frees herself from the Ahrimanic error.

As we said, most of the women whose cancer is detected at an early stage will recover. This means stopping the disease at its onset. Thus in fact the woman is prevented from having at least part of the experiences that were supposed to afford the development requested by her spiritual being. However, the treatment itself, the surgery, the chemotherapy and the radiation, and the ongoing fears of death and separation, all constitute a considerable load of experiences that are not at all easy. From this point of view, even the current process of the disease, which begins with early detection and ends in recovery, gives the person's soul the possibility to grow through hardships. In fact, no one walks along this path without it leaving its mark on his soul.

However, just as the person's spiritual being does not

always succeed in accomplishing its objectives fully through a serious disease, the same is true when the disease is prevented or the person recovers from it. The spiritual development of the person is slow and ridden with obstacles. It is possible that the early detection of a disease and its prevention are liable to constitute an additional obstacle along the human being's path of development. A weakness from one incarnation that is not strengthened in the second incarnation will assume a clearer expression, perhaps in the form of a disability, in the third incarnation.

Healing has always been a mystery. The person does everything in his power to recover. He is assisted by the best physicians and the most advanced technologies, he sees that he supplies his body with all the necessary vitamins and minerals, and he approaches healers, therapists and support groups that can reinforce his soul. Even so, healing is not a foregone conclusion. The person's earthly consciousness leads him to do everything in order to recover, and in this way mobilizes itself unconsciously to serve his spiritual aims as well. Today, as at any other time, the person's spiritual being, which aspires to the good, is the one that directs his destiny.

After doing everything possible, there is nothing left to do but to resign oneself. Illness is the person's great teacher. Through it, he can learn to accept his life as it is and forgive his own weaknesses. He can rejoice in every sunbeam and rediscover the beauty of the waves rolling to the shore. Through the disease, he can wake up to the love he feels for people. The person who has made peace with himself will have the strength to accept anything destiny deals him. In his very lifetime, his earthly consciousness is getting closer to his spiritual consciousness. Goodness touches him and, through him, the people around him as well.

The sick person is accompanied by family and friends who do everything they can for him. Sometimes their loved one recovers and sometimes he doesn't. A person who loses someone close, a person who is forced to separate from a dear one, can perhaps find a little consolation if he pays attention to what Anthroposophy says about it. People naturally tend to view their loss through a heavy screen of mourning and pain. However, if they allow the spiritual thoughts of the karma to resonate in their souls over time, they are likely to gradually penetrate the screen and reach the point where they recognize the development their dear one went through. When a person can see death not only from a subjective point of view but also from the objective point of view of the spirit, it becomes a source of solace and strength for him.

From the point of view of the soul that has crossed the threshold to the world of the soul, the manner in which the people near to it in the physical world view its situation is of particularly great significance. In most cases, a person who is in the physical world on this side of the threshold of death is incapable of directly experiencing someone who has crossed the threshold of the worlds of soul and spirit. The person who died becomes a memory for him. Memory, because of its own nature, is a mental image that is complete in itself. While the memory can be extremely painful and dear and fill the person's soul, it has no possibility of renewal except in the sanctification of the past. In contrast, the human being who has separated from his physical body and finds himself in the world of the soul feels the people who are connected to him in a more intimate way. Since the body no longer poses a barrier for him, he experiences the souls of those close to him from inside. The feelings and thoughts, pain and happiness of those who were dear to him in his life are obvious to him after his death just as their external appearance was obvious to him before his death. When the soul of a human being who died identifies spiritual thoughts in the heart of the living person, it experiences a feeling that can be compared to what a person in the physical world feels when he gains the attention of a person close to him. He knows that the person close to him in the living world acknowledges his existence now. Spiritual thoughts in the heart of someone close illuminate the path of the soul that has gone over the threshold of death into the worlds of soul and spirit[26].

The state of medicine

Medicine between Lucifer and Ahriman

The treatment of breast cancer, as described in the previous chapter, is an example of the level of sophistication of advanced medicine. It contains diverse techniques that belong to various fields of medicine: surgery, chemotherapy, radiation, and hormonal treatment. What all these have in common is the fact that they are directed at the patient's physical body. Hospitals nowadays also employ social workers and psychologists whose job it is to speak to the patient and assist him in everything that is beyond the physical level. However, all those good people and the perceptions they represent are not an integral part of medicine itself. Western medicine relates to the disease as if it were a breakdown in the person's physical mechanism that has to be repaired, and the value of everything around it is measured according to its direct effect on the physical condition. The physician is interested in the patient's profession if it exposes him to the causes of the disease – to carcinogenic substances, for instance. He is interested in the patient's family if there are other family members with the same disease, because he can then assume that there is a hereditary tendency involved. Will the person's family be able to support him and care for him after his release from hospital? Is the person looking forward to the moment he can return to work, or does that moment spark deep anxiety in him? These questions, which shape the entire world of the person who has fallen ill and now has to muster the strength for the recovery process, are ignored in the state-of-the-art medical system surrounding the patient.

One of the most worn-out pictures used by critics of the medical system is that of the doctors' rounds, which take place on a daily basis in every hospital ward. All the physicians in the department – their numbers can reach a dozen or more – go from one bed to the next. The physicians discuss the condition of the patient lying in the bed among themselves; sometimes they palpate his abdomen or listen to his chest, thank him politely and move on. The ideal patient, according to the prevailing patronizing attitude in the halls of modern medicine, is obedient and passive. He lies quietly and does not make trouble. In the meantime, the soul of the person who is lying in the hospital bed and listening to his ailment being discussed is completely shrouded in a feeling of alienation and foreignness. Many of the physicians who work in the hospitals and clinics are devoted doctors who consider every person's dignity and feelings to be more important than anything else. However, the force that separates people and causes the feeling of alienation is stronger than they are. That is the Ahrimanic influence that motivates advanced medicine on the one hand and threatens to destroy any human contact that may still exist in it on the other.

A person who has contracted a serious disease is seeking warmth, human closeness and a sympathetic ear for his distress – especially after his encounter with the official medical system. One of the possibilities open to him is that of joining a support group. All over the Western world, people who suffer from a particular disease – or people who have a family member with the disease – have gotten organized and begun to meet. During these meetings, the sick person may well learn about solutions to problems he has run into from people in a similar situation. He can share his fears with people who are carrying the same burden and he can give and receive human warmth. Over the years, scientific research on the topic of support groups has been conducted, proving that they have an effect on the mental domain. People who availed themselves of these groups – especially those whose anxiety levels were high from the start – suffered less from anxiety as compared with people who did not avail themselves of the groups. They also suffered less from pain. These two effects belong to the mental domain. In contrast, in the domain of overcoming the disease, at least according to the research that has been conducted on people with cancer, it seems that the support groups do not have an advantage. In other words, the experience of support and human warmth does not exert a real effect on the physical condition[27].

People who are seeking a more personal relationship than what exists in the official system frequently turn to healers. One of the reasons that "psychic healing" of various kinds is widespread is because it does not conflict with any conventional medical treatment and therefore does not bother the physicians. We have already mentioned that "psychic healing" is not in the person's control, but rather it is a rare phenomenon that can occur between two people who are connected by a special karmic connection. When "healing" becomes an income-generating occupation, it is usually after the healing forces have been used up. What the various kinds of individual or group treatments have in common is the good feeling the patient has at the end of the treatment. The good feeling stems precisely from the element in the person's soul that is reinforced by the intimate encounter with another person or other people. As in support groups, the anxiety level drops and the loneliness is less acute.

The external force the person encounters via conventional medicine is the force of Ahriman. The internal force the person encounters after receiving the "positive energy" from an individual or a group is the force of Lucifer. The conventional medical treatments cope, sometimes successfully, with the physical disease, but they do not have access to the person's spiritual and soul being. The "energies" that flow from one person to the next affect the recipient's soul, sometimes to the point of intoxication, but they cannot penetrate the sick organs. Like the whole of humanity and like every individual, medicine, too, is facing the challenge of creating a connection between the poles, of finding the golden path between matter and spirit, between outside and inside, between Ahriman and Lucifer.

Arrogance and suppression

It would be a mistake to think that the Luciferic temptation operates via complementary or alternative medicine alone, and that the Ahrimanic error is only evident in the medicine of the natural sciences. Like the diseases of the era, it is possible to identify both influences in all the medical trends of our times. Arrogance, for example, accompanies scientific breakthroughs that promise to liberate the human species from every kind of illness. That same arrogance is also revealed in all kinds of miracle preparations or all-curing instruments that pop up in the periphery of alternative medicine. Amazing new methods for the fast and easy cure of too many illnesses reach us regularly from all corners of the world. Among them are fastidious diets that claim to cure cancer, potions for fortifying the immune system that claim to have an effect on cancer, AIDS and a series of other diseases, and laser instruments that heal all joint and skeletal pains with no need to find out what is causing them. Many people, therapists and patients alike, are easily convinced to believe in these methods, which actually do help in certain situations. It is only when people begin to believe in their omnipotence that the problems arise. While many people are convinced, many more – and not just professional people, but also anyone who uses his common sense – realize that these are nothing but futile claims. In contrast, when it is a matter of real scientific innovations that are accompanied by a media circus, even logical people are taken in.

The scientific achievements themselves are good and

effective. Antibiotics, for instance, which constituted the outstanding achievement of the second half of the twentieth century, saved many people from death. However, the promise made by the researchers fifty years ago – namely, that all the infectious diseases would disappear from the world – was not kept. The bacteria become resistant, unknown bacteria appear, and people still continue their soul and spiritual development by means of diseases as in days gone by. We have already mentioned the ambitious plans to rid the world of diseases by means of global immunization, as well as the widespread battle to prevent the birth of babies with hereditary diseases. What happened in parallel was the appearance of new diseases at the same time as the old ones were eliminated, and a rise of hundreds of percent in the number of babies with developmental disorders that can only be identified when the child has already been born. All these demonstrate the futility of human technology when it is directed with enthusiastic ignorance against the laws of the world of the spirit that guide the development of humanity. It must be reiterated and stressed that the aspiration to eradicate a disease like smallpox, which caused so much suffering, from human destiny, is noble. However, when targeting human destiny, it is impossible to make do with considerations from the field of viral science or any other physical and biological consideration. It is essential to relate to the whole human being in order to understand how it is really possible to influence the destiny of humankind today, so that our deeds will not come back at us like a boomerang.

The latest scientific breakthrough is the deciphering of the human genome, a great achievement that will engender the development of new and effective medications. Like the previous achievements, however, it will not put an end to human suffering either. It is another opportunity for arrogance to make a big splash in all the media and prove that humanity, which has developed a worshipful attitude toward science since the nineteenth century, does not learn from experience. Of course there is a reason for this. The human being still perceives the world around him as a hostile and dangerous place that threatens his health and life. Scientific achievements provide him with the illusion that he will soon be in control of his life and will finally be able to harness the powers of creation to serve him.

When we shift our gaze from the general development of medicine to its cornerstone – the intimate encounter between physician and patient – exactly the same forces are found there. Arrogance, as many people know from their own experience, even if they did not call it by that name, is one of the physician's most common defense mechanisms. The very young and intellectually gifted person who decides to study medicine out of idealism, is exposed to a great deal of knowledge during the course of his studies. He acquires the ability to apply a large number of diagnostic and therapeutic methods and sets out along his professional path enthusiastically. On the outside, in the real world, however, a reality for which he has not been prepared awaits him. Already in his first encounters with the destinies of sick people, the young person's soul experiences the pain of his inability to offer the person in front of him genuine succor. His soul undergoes a partially conscious process of wising up. It begins to understand that the tremendous body of knowledge it has acquired sheds no light on the person's spiritual and soul being. Then, in an attempt to protect himself against his lack of knowledge and his impotence, the physician cloaks himself in the shining armor of arrogance. It is important to mention once more that there are also many doctors for whom humility is an inseparable part of their personalities and of the way in which they deal with their patients. And still, in Western society, young people with good intellectual abilities have a monopoly of medical studies. Because the academic medical establishment is blind to anything concerning the person's soul and spirit, it does almost nothing to try to identify the people with wisdom of the heart among those clamoring at its doors.

Arrogance gives the physician an illusion of protection against overly close contact with reality and with sick people and their destinies. Suppression performs the same service for the sick person himself. People whose lives have been invaded by illness – even if a kind of prescience or undefined fear nested beforehand in the depths of their consciousness – still experience their new situation as a total shock. The disease is accompanied by pain, physical and mental limitations, and the fear of death. For anyone who lives his entire life without consciously asking about the meaning of his life, without seeking the spiritual in the world, the very thought of approaching death is unbearably difficult. Suppression serves the person's fear of coping with his destiny with eyes wide open. The use the sick person makes of this mental defense mechanism also solves a problem for the physician, who wants to avoid the deep emotional involvement that is required for a frank and genuine conversation with his patient.

The following example depicts a very common situation. People who have cancer that has already spread from its initial location and has metastasized to other organs generally receive chemotherapy whose objective is to decrease the amount of cancerous cells in their body and give them a certain period of time in which the disease remains dormant. The doctors know that only in a few instances does this treatment eliminate the cancer. However, when the course of treatment ends and the patient fearfully asks what is supposed to happen, the common answer is: "You're healthy now, you've got nothing to worry about." The logic behind this answer is that in any case, medicine has no more effective treatments to offer the person at this stage, so there is no point exposing him to the likelihood that the disease will return. When that happens, additional chemotherapy or radiation treatment may be considered, but it is no use jumping the gun.

The physician in the described scene signals to the patient what his preferred extent of frankness in the dialog between them is. He opens the door to suppression for the patient. The very fact of passing through the door and deciding to close his eyes to reality is already the patient's choice – and not always a conscious one. There are people who reject the possibility of suppression that the doctor offers them and turn, at this juncture of their lives, to other places for help and healing. Not surprisingly, they can encounter the same principle of suppression among the various methods of complementary medicine. This mental defense mechanism can also hide behind techniques such as "positive thinking" – a method that can in itself be beneficial.

In this method, the person is directed to fill his consciousness with positive and optimistic contents, and not to deal with his illness and fears. The chapter, "Consciousness and healing", described the person's ability to imbue a state of chronic illness with tranquillity and stability by focusing his consciousness on new contents instead of dwelling on pain and fear. Such a process can only occur in a person who is completely aware of his condition, and decides to expend the forces of his soul on positive action in spite of it. It will never occur in a person who is afraid to look his illness in the eye and uses positive thoughts like heavy stones that he piles up at the entrance of the cave from which the truth threatens to break out at any moment.

How to heal medicine

In the past, a person was born in a certain place – a village or a suburb – and lived his entire life there. Many of his human ties lasted for decades. This was also true of his relationship with his physician. The physician accompanied his aged parents until they died and treated his children's fever ilnesses. Today, the situation is different. The Western welfare states take care of funding the medical services of even the poorest of their citizens by means of medical insurance mechanisms. Thanks to the public health organizations, many people from the weaker strata have been provided with a more or less orderly approach to medical services. However, progress has not only brought advantages. It has also led to the severing of the personal relationship between patient and doctor. Today, when a person needs medical care, he does not go to a physician, but rather to a clinic, an emergency room, or to companies that provide medical services. He turns to an organization, not to a person.

Within the medical establishment, too, people yearn for the human touch that modern medicine has lost. Physicians with a humanistic attitude try to bolster family medicine and restore the old framework of long-term, quality ties between patient and doctor. Physicians participate in workshops for interpersonal relations. They learn to look at themselves and identify their own private fears so that they can prevent them from sneaking into their encounter with the patient. However, this "humanistic" attitude is still not central in medicine. These contents must become an inseparable part of the training of every doctor, and not just the training of general practitioners in community clinics. The medical establishment has to understand what is ostensibly self-evident: first and foremost, the physician must learn to be a "person". His professional-technical knowledge, important as it might be, is of secondary importance.

Nevertheless, even when this happens, it will be impossible to restore the old ties between patient and doctor. The world has changed, and along with it, human encounters have also changed. People move from rural to urban areas and back, from country to country, change professions, divorce and remarry. They are more mobile and less bound by social conventions. The change in modern life reflects changes in human karma. The contemporary person has acquired connections with many human beings in his previous incarnations, and he continues to process all these connections in his present life as well. The result of this karmic complexity may be that the encounters between people nowadays are relatively short but more intense than acquaintances that endured a lifetime in the past. This is also true for the encounter between patient and doctor. Sometimes, a person can meet the doctor a few times or even once; something happens to him as a result of the encounter, and his life changes. Let's take a person who suffers from an allergy to some kind of food. The physician discovers the cause of the allergy by means of the questions he asks the patient or by means of tests, and instructs the person to refrain from eating that particular food. Sometimes, that is enough to get rid of the allergic phenomena that have plagued the person for years. Another person, who suffers from recurrent attacks of back pains, discovers the link between the pains and the profound dissatisfaction he has experienced in his work for years as a result of the doctor's questions.

The physician can also learn from every encounter with a patient, even if it only lasts a few minutes. Every physician remembers encounters that caused him to change the way he relates to people, the way he perceives his job as a doctor, or even his professional direction. Encounters of the type described are not coincidental or random. They are encounters that belong to the person's karma. In the ties between patient and doctor – and this holds true for nurses and therapists as well – one person asks another person to help him live his life. In other words, the person asks his fellow human being to intervene with his karma. Every doctor or therapist intervenes in the destinies of the people who come to him for treatment, even if he meets them during his night shift in the hospital or is simply standing in for the regular general practitioner for half a day.

Because of the limitations of human consciousness, people today are unable to be aware of the effects their actions have on other people's karma or on their own karma. If people were aware of the spiritual significance of every action they perform, every thought they think or every feeling they feel, they would relate to the meeting with another person with great awe. Ostensibly, there is no need to accept and believe in the existence of a spiritual reality in order to understand that if humility were to take the place of arrogance, and courage were to push fear out of the person's soul, medicine would be more human once again. This is not the case, however. Over the years, physicians with a humanistic approach that is not supported by a spiritual world view, lose the enthusiasm and the belief they had at the beginning of their careers. They find themselves competing for jobs and money, administering unnecessary treatments in order not to become embroiled in lawsuits, writing medical reports and doing a thousand things that have no bearing on healing the sick person.

The materialistic world view, which so flatters the human intellect, cannot nourish the deep layers of the soul. It has spawned a reality that has no place for the person – neither the patient nor the therapist. At the beginning of the twenty first century, a person who asks an existential question finds himself poised at the edge of a dark abyss with no way across it. Only if the person acknowledges the existence of the spirit and acknowledges himself to be a spiritual being, can he get a true response to his fear of the dark around him.

That is the great secret of the future. When human culture again acknowledges the person as a being that comes from the spiritual world, medicine, too, will stop being detached and alien. The reader is liable to feel disappointed with the remedy offered here for healing medicine. He may claim that such changes in consciousness will happen in the distant future, if they happen at all, and this leaves humanity with a difficult problem in the present. This worry seems to be justified, but there are places in which the seeds of future consciousness have already been planted. These seeds are found in every action taken by a person out of a sense of idealism, in every deed a person does for another person. One of the fields that borders on medicine, in which not only are the seeds of the future sown, but it is already possible to find an acknowledgment of the person as a spiritual being, is curative education. This is the name given to the work with children with special needs that began in the 1920s, when several educators and physicians turned to Rudolf Steiner and requested his guidance.

Curative education is based on the perception of the person as a being that consists of a spiritual "I", a soul body, a life body and a physical body. Many of the children with special needs have a certain weakness in their life body. Normally, each one of the person's bodies develops under the influence of the one above it. That is, the "I" forms the soul body, the soul body forms the life body, and so on. In order to achieve a curative effect on the life body of the child with special needs, the educator must make use of his own soul body. In other words, the educator knows that in order to achieve any kind of progress, he must first educate his own soul body. Only in this way will he be able to achieve a true and constant effect on the child's life body[28].

At first sight, this can remind us of what has been said about "psychic healing". There, too, we spoke about the effect that flows from one person to another. However, there are essential differences between the two phenomena. "Psychic healing" is based on an effect that is transmitted from one person to another in an instinctive manner, that is, without any control on the part of the "healer" over what is happening. In contrast, the curative educator spends years making a conscious effort to turn himself into a vehicle of healing forces. The "healing" can only occur when there is an exceptional karmic connection between two people, while the crux of the self-education of the educator is meant to overcome the subjective element in the relationship between him and the children. The educator can only reach the child after he has paved the way between the sympathy and the antipathy he feels toward him. Then he can effect a healing, sometimes small, sometimes big, for each child, without any dependence on the personal relationship between them.

Any person who develops consciousness of his self and aspires to transform himself in order to help others, acquires humility over time. Anyone who works with children out of such consciousness knows that with his paltry forces he is affecting their spiritual being; in other words, he is intervening with their destiny. A person who consciously operates like that develops courage. Thanks to courage and humility, small triumphs over arrogance and fear occur daily in dozens of curative education communities spread over five continents. In such places, the way is paved for guiding humanity and along with it, medicine, toward the future. And who is leading humanity along the path to the future? The children who require curative education, those same children who suffer from disabilities or abuse. By the very fact of their fragile and vulnerable existence among the rest of us, they give humanity the most valuable gift of all – the possibility to act out of love.

Spiritual training

Discretion

Although a description of spiritual training does not belong directly to the topic of illness and healing, it is appropriate to provide a brief overview of the anthroposophic spiritual path. After all, it is through spiritual experience that the point of view of destiny is revealed to human consciousness. All the descriptions of supersensible reality that are quoted in the book stem from the works of Rudolf Steiner, and they were achieved by direct spiritual experience. The chapter is brief and limited and cannot serve as a practical guide for training. Anyone who truly aspires to work toward achieving direct experience of the spiritual world is advised to invest his time in a careful study of books that were written first-hand and especially for this purpose[1].

Even before a person does some conscious deed in order to achieve a spiritual experience, he has to examine what is motivating him to want such an experience. A person who desires to gain spiritual knowledge in order to exploit it for his own personal benefit in some way can expect to be bitterly disappointed. The higher spiritual beings to whom the person's soul is revealed will not enable a person with selfish motives to enter the world of the spirit, even if he himself is completely unaware of the forces at work in his soul. In our context, even the aspiration to achieve spiritual knowledge and use it in order to cure a disease cannot help the person cope with the difficult tests that every pupil of a true spiritual path has to face. Only a person who wishes to learn how he can serve the world better will receive the help of the higher beings. The path to the spirit, by its very nature, does not promise anything but a change of consciousness to the person who follows it.

Many books have been written about the path to spiritual experience and the attainment of spiritual knowledge. Some of them are based on true knowledge of the spiritual world, but some are not. There is a simple yardstick that can help us begin the task of differentiating between the two types of books. We can generalize and say that any book that promises a fast and easy path to spiritual experiences or to encounters with spiritual beings belongs to the realm of charlatanism. Books that offer rapid spiritual development, as well as weekend workshops that promise their participants the ability to see auras, are no different from miracle potions or treatments that claim to cure serious diseases without any effort on the part of the patient. Every knowledgeable person knows that in order to play the piano well it is necessary to practice and persevere for years. Knowledge of the spiritual world is also attained through perseverance. So much for the "instant" methods and books for spiritual development, but the deceptions do not end here. Not every book that describes spiritual development as a path that is fraught with difficulties and pitfalls, is necessarily a reliable guide to the spiritual world. In other words, even after the preliminary sifting, there are still many books by people who indeed attained spiritual experiences, but the direction they suggest does not have any value beyond their private karmic context.

In the last decades, more people are succeeding in attaining spiritual experiences of various kinds[29]. One example of such experiences is that of clinical death. Most of the clinical death experiences that have been described are limited, even though for the person involved in them, they are extremely powerful. In contrast, George Ritchie's experience, which was extraordinary in its dimensions, is of real value to anyone who reads about it, and not just for the person who experienced it. Ritchie's experience gives a broad picture of the world of the soul, while the other clinical death experiences simply stand on its threshold. Like clinical death experiences, other spiritual experiences also differ from one another in their extent and significance. Most of them have direct value mainly for the person who experiences them, but not for humanity in general. Not every supersensible experience turns the person who had it into a spiritual teacher, since most of them do not even come near to experiencing the infinite wealth of the spiritual world. There are very few people whose knowledge of the spiritual world is profound to a degree that enables them to show others the path to spiritual experience and assume full responsibility for the consequences of their directions.

One of the problems that is liable to arise as a result of directions for spiritual training being given by people with only a partial knowledge of the spiritual world is the undermining of the mental stability of sensitive people. A spiritual teacher can only be someone who can implement the required preventive measures in order to prevent young people from engaging in any practice that is liable to make the ground collapse beneath their feet. The person who brought Anthroposophy into the world at the beginning of the twentieth century, Rudolf Steiner, was identified by some of his contemporaries as one of the great teachers of humanity. The directions for spiritual training that appear in his books and in his lectures are always accompanied by explanations and are never arbitrary. They were written with the aim of helping the pupil maintain his mental equilibrium every step of the way. We have already mentioned the uniqueness of Anthroposophy among other spiritual movements. This is reflected in the fact that it addresses independent thinking and lucid consciousness. Particularly when it comes to taking up a spiritual training, there is no substitute for the person's own discretion.

About meditation and the necessary preparation for it

A person who aspires to create healing forces in his soul can do so by immersing himself in the image of sunlight, as was described in the chapter on self-healing. This spiritual and soul process, which has a healing effect on the life body, is called meditation. The word *meditation* is used today to describe states and activities that can be very different than or even opposed to one another. The repetition of certain sounds that is customary in Hindi, Buddhist and other methods is called meditation, as are the techniques of concentrating on breathing or on other physical processes that are also widespread in the East.

Even physical and mental relaxation exercises can appear under the heading of meditation. Meditation comes from a Latin word that is connected to the Western spiritual tradition and describes a process of immersing oneself in spiritual contents, of praying or of contemplating religious or philosophical thoughts, accompanied by the detachment of the human soul from the world of the senses. Even this definition can still contain a broad range of diverse activities.

The aim of this brief introduction is in fact to ask the reader to free himself, at least temporarily, from all his preconceptions regarding meditation so that the contents offered by Anthroposophy for this spiritual and soul activity can resonate in his soul.

How is meditation performed? The person must find a time and a place in which he can cut himself off from any contact with the world around him. He must make sure that freeing up this time does not come at the expense of his everyday commitments. After creating the circumstances that ensure physical and mental tranquillity, he should sit comfortably so that the position does not distract him from the matter at hand. The Western person is usually accustomed to sitting on a chair. Now he must place a suitable content at the center of his consciousness and concentrate all of his soul forces on it. This content can be a thought, an idea or a pictorial image of a spiritual truth. The thought about spiritual existence taking precedence over physical existence is an example of this kind of content. The same is true for the picture of the sunlight that fills the person's soul and body, which is a suitable image of the healing force that flows from the spiritual world. In anthroposophic literature, there are many contents that can be used for meditation. Initially, at least, it is advisable to choose images that are not too complex, since it is easier to concentrate on them.

The meditation process described involves all of the person's soul forces. In everyday life, human thinking is filled with all the contents that come to it from the outside. The person himself has almost no control over what is occupying his thoughts. In meditation, on the other hand, human thinking is asked to concentrate on content that is not forced on it from the outside. This content has a more delicate texture than any of the other thoughts human thinking is used to – the ones that are linked to objects and occurrences in the physical world. Human feelings are also involved in meditation. In normal life, the person is even less in control of his feelings than he is of his thoughts. In meditation, however the feelings, too, must concentrate on the chosen image and slowly and gradually turn into a kind of sense organ by means of which the person can touch the spiritual reality at whose doors he is knocking. Mobilizing the thinking and taming the feelings cannot be accomplished without the full and constant involvement of the third soul force, the will.

The reinforcement of the three soul forces is a prerequisite in order for meditation to lead to spiritual cognition. In addition, the person also has to examine carefully to what extent he is controlled by prejudices or various iron-clad principles that are liable to prevent the germination of spiritual truths in his soul right at the outset. A critical attitude toward the world and adherence to rigid standpoints cool and harden the soul. Spiritual cognition, in contrast, can only develop in a soul that is imbued with life and warmth. It has already been said that the description of meditation presented here is deliberately extremely brief. Anyone who really wants to take the long and arduous path of spiritual training is well advised to do some attentive preliminary reading, particularly regarding the conditions and preparation required for meditation[30].

In most cases, when the person closes his eyes and detaches his attention from the world of the senses, he does not experience anything at first. Meditation requires a great deal of persistence. It is actually a process in which the person grows supersensible sense organs in his soul body and his life body. These organs are able to perceive the spiritual world as the eye and the ear perceive the physical world. However, long before the person acquires the ability to perceive the spiritual world, he can already feel the delicate and significant changes that occur inside him during meditation. He is still cloaked in darkness, but inside him he can feel a kind of expanse that is revealing itself in his soul, an expanse that is stirring with life despite the darkness. The spiritual thoughts the person has placed at the center of his consciousness now become living beings. They are different than the thoughts that serve him in the world of the senses, which are perceived by him as shadows that are cast by physical reality. We can understand the change if we recall the clinical death experience once more. A person who has had this experience sees the entire picture of his life revealed to him as a result of the detachment of his higher bodies from his physical body. His physical senses do not respond to him and he sees around him what has been collected and preserved in his life body all his life. Going back to the person who is meditating, whose soul feels the dark and life-filled expanse and the harmonious movement of the thoughts that occur in him, this too is a primal experience of one's own life body. Since there is no detachment of the physical body from the life body in this case, the experience remains dark and does not reach the stage of a real spiritual vision. The time for the latter will only come when the higher worlds find the person strong enough and ready to pass through their gates.

On the threshold of the world of the spirit

According to Rudolf Steiner's descriptions, the person who perseveres with spiritual training undergoes many wondrous experiences. We will mention two of them, which, for quite a few contemporary people, are not so distant and fantastic. These two experiences meet the person even before he crosses the threshold of the spiritual world, and they are both universal. This means that today it is not possible to attain an actual experience of the spiritual world in a voluntary and controlled manner without being exposed in one way or another to both of them.

Along the path to spiritual knowledge, the person learns to know himself. He is exposed to his innate selfishness and to the gnawing doubt in his heart. However, at a certain point, after he has already acquired a measure of mental strength, a terrible image is revealed to him. It accompanies him and he finds no refuge from it. The pupil discovers himself in this distorted image. It is the negative side of his being; all of his weaknesses are expressed in it, as is all the evil he has caused in the world. Before the gates of the spiritual world are thrown open to him, the pupil has to redeem the image that accompanies him – which is in fact himself – from the monstrous ugliness. He must persevere and develop his morality until this distorted image no longer exists.

Then, on the very threshold of the spiritual world, a being of infinite love and light awaits him. We already know this being from the descriptions of clinical death experiences, from the revelations experienced by mystics in the past, and even from experiences that people have during the course of their regular lives today. Now and then it happens that people who are in great distress and pray for salvation from the depths of their soul experience the being of light and are granted consolation. From the day this being of infinite love touches their souls, the way they perceive their lives and the world changes completely. This being also places itself in front of the person who wishes to enter the spiritual world in order to protect him from entering it prematurely. A person who has prepared himself and is able to enter the world of the spirit and also return from it whole in soul and spirit has the privilege of passing through the gate[31].

The two experiences described above take us back to illness and healing. The distorted image is the sum total of the person's weaknesses and flaws. It arouses the person who consciously aspires to the spiritual world to take action to correct his weaknesses. The people who are sick with serious diseases overcome the weaknesses of their soul through life itself.

The being of infinite love and light is the source of all the healing forces that flowed in the past and that will flow in the future from the world of the spirit to humanity. The more the spiritual world occupies a place in the person's everyday consciousness, the more the kindness and healing that shine from it on to the world of the senses will become an actual experience for him.

Notes and bibliography

All of the books or lecture series that appear without the author's name are the works of Rudolf Steiner. Some of these books are published by two or more publishers under different titles. The main publishers of Rudolf Steiner's works in the English language are Rudolf Steiner Press in the U.K and SteinerBooks or Anthroposophic Press in the U.S.A.

1. The description of the path to a direct supersensible experience appears in the book: *How to Know Higher Worlds*, SteinerBooks (also published as: *Knowledge of the Higher Worlds*, Rudolf Steiner Press). A comprehensive chapter on spiritual development also appears in the book: *An Outline of Esoteric Science*, SteinerBooks.

2. A description of the process of cognition that forms the basis of the anthroposophic world-view can be found in the book: *Intuitive Thinking as a Spiritual Path; A Philosophy of Freedom*, SteinerBooks (also published as: *The Philosophy of Freedom*, Rudolf Steiner Press).

3. More can be read about the life body in particular and the whole human being in general in the following books: *Theosophy*, SteinerBooks, and: *An Outline of Esoteric Science*, SteinerBooks. These are two of the fundamental books of Anthroposophy. With regard to the training that leads to supersensible experience, see Note #1.

4. The names chosen here to indicate the supersensible components of the human being are not the only ones that exist nor are they necessarily the best. The life body is better known in occult traditions as the etheric body, and the soul body is better known as the astral body. In anthroposophic literature, the first is sometimes called the body of formative forces and the second the sentient body. The terms "life body" and "soul body" are preferred because they are simpler and perhaps relatively free from preconceptions. The main shortcoming of the term "soul body" is the fact that it may be confused with the soul itself, which is created from the interaction of the "I" with all the bodies, and not just with the soul body. The soul body is still the main vehicle of the person's experience of self and so it is not a mistake to call it by this name. More about the human soul in the subsection: "Spirit and soul come first".

5. The relationship between the human being and the four elements is discussed in the following lecture series: *The Bridge between Universal Spirituality and the Physical Constitution of Man*, Anthroposophic Press.

6. More about waking and sleeping in the book: *An Outline of Esoteric Science*, SteinerBooks.

7. The experience of soul and spirit that is born in the person's consciousness is described from another angle in the subsection, "Meditation and the necessary preparation for it". Numerous examples of meditative exercises can be found in the book: *How to Know Higher Worlds*, SteinerBooks.

8. Raymond A. Moodie's book: *Life after Life*, contains a survey of a series of reports on clinical death experiences. George Ritchie's experience is described in his book: *Returning from Tomorrow.*

9. More about life after death can be found in the fundamental books mentioned in Note #3.

10. More about the evolution of humanity and the earth can be found in: *An Outline of Esoteric Science*, SteinerBooks, and in: *Cosmic Memory*, Garber Books.

11. The lecture series that deals with karma in general and the karma of illnesses in particular is: *Manifestation of Karma*, Rudolf Steiner Press. An introduction to the understanding of karma also appears in the fundamental books listed in Note #3.

12. For an expansion on the topic of febrile illnesses and childrens health in general see: Goebel and Glockler, *A Guide to Child Health*, Floris Books .

13. For more about cancer, see: Murphy (ed.), *Iscador: Mistletoe and Cancer Therapy*, Lantern Books.

14. While the smallpox virus no longer exists as a cause of disease in nature, it still threatens the safety of humanity. After its extinction from nature, the virus has been preserved in research laboratories, and some people fear that it will fall into the wrong hands and be used as a biological weapon one day. If this ever happens, it is liable to be particularly dangerous because the general public is no longer vaccinated against it.

15. Sensory deprivation as a cause of birth defects in the next incarnation is described in the first lecture of: *Education for Special Needs*, Rudolf Steiner Press.

16. *Manifestation of Karma*, Rudolf Steiner Press.

17. The claims supporting or denying a link between the MMR [measles, mumps, rubella] vaccination and autism appear in many articles in the medical literature as well as in the regular press. A great deal of material on this topic can be found in the archives of the websites of the various media.

18. The fact that women today no longer devote themselves only to the traditional domains of the family and the children may be linked to the fact that painless birth is a possibility today. The phenomenon that is called "women's liberation" is the fruit of the evolving self-consciousness of women, which legitimizes the fulfillment of the woman's needs rather than just being at the beck and call of her husband and children. This is an example of how the Luciferic influence contributes to the development of human consciousness.

19. The self-healing process as well as the "psychic healing" process are described in the lecture series for medical students: *Course for Young Doctors*, Mercury Press. With regard to diseases of the soul body and the life body as opposed to diseases of the physical body: a phenomenon such as "irritable bowel syndrome", which is expressed in stomach pains and digestive difficulties, but reveals no findings in imaging examinations of the digestive organs, is an example of a disorder in the relationship between the soul body and the life body in the intestinal region. In contrast, when there is evidence of a real inflammatory process in the intestinal wall, such as ulcerative colitis or Crohn's disease, it indicates a disease that has descended to the physical body. Another common example comes from the respiratory system. Smoking initially causes a disorder in the relationship between the soul body and the life body, a disorder that is reversible if one stops smoking. If one continues, the effect of smoking can penetrate the physical structure of the lungs and assume forms of a chronic inflammation, sometimes leading to cancer.

20. Christ acts of healing are described by Rudolf Steiner in a series of lectures called: *The Gospel of St. Luke*, Rudolf Steiner Press.

21. Why make unnecessary use of medications? Here are some of the many answers that exist to this complex question: With regard to cancer patients who are receiving chemotherapy that is not effective for their disease, the reason is the physicians' desire to do *something*, no matter what. They do not want to abandon the patient to his fate without treatment, so they treat him in the way they know. Sometimes the patient and his family force the oncologist to administer the treatment against his better judgment. Not only oncologists, but also pediatricians frequently prescribe medications that go against medical considerations because of the pressure exerted on them by the child's parents. We refer, for instance, to antibiotics that are prescribed in the case of a viral infection. Another reason for unnecessary treatments in general – not just regarding medications – is the physicians' fear of lawsuits. One of the most blatant examples is the great increase in the percentage of infants delivered by Caesarean section. These operations are sometimes performed even when there is no medical justification for them. If any problem arises, the doctor can claim that he did the maximum – surgery, in this case – to prevent it. Coming back to the unnecessary use of medications, we must not forget the decisive contribution of the gigantic drug companies to this practice. It will not be an overstatement to say that the drug manufacturers do not reject any marketing strategy that will get physicians to prescribe their medications – the more the merrier.

22. Regarding the use of natural medications from an anthroposophic point of view, see: Husemann/Wolff,

Anthroposophical Approach to Medicine, SteinerBooks. This book is meant for physicians and medical students. A more popular book by Otto Wolff is *Home Remedies*, SteinerBooks.

23. Besides the above-mentioned examples, the most obvious example for the "quality blindness" of nutritional science is its indifference to the issue of chemical substances in food. The studies that attempt to link agricultural pesticides of various kinds that are found in food to diseases also encounter the difficulty of proving the link between two phenomena that may be far away from each other in time. Moreover, it is difficult to isolate the exposure to chemical substances via food from the exposure via air pollution and water and soil pollution. However, the link of chemical pollution of various kinds to serious illness has already been proved beyond a doubt, for example by studies that found a much higher prevalence of malignancies of the blood, nervous system and urinary tract among farmers and others exposed to pesticides. Other statistics that support this link show an increase in cancer rates in several heavily industrialized areas around the globe in comparison to non-industrialised regions.

24. The anthroposophic point of view regarding the physical, soul and spiritual development of the human being is described in Bernard Lievegoed's book: *Phases*, Rudolf Steiner Press.

25. Biographical contemplation can be done independently by anyone who has studied and knows the spiritual and soul development of the human being. In the context of treating a sick person, "biographical counselling" is generally done with the help of a therapist or a doctor.

26. In the lecture: *The Dead Are with Us*, Rudolf Steiner Press, the way in which the soul experiences the world of the soul and the spirit after death is described. It also describes how people can communicate with the human beings that are close to them who have passed over the threshold of death, without falling into dangerous illusions. The kind of communication that is described is completely different than anything that is known as mediumistic phenomena. In Dore Deverell's book, *Light Beyond the Darkness*, Temple Lodge, an event involving the formation of a connection between two individuals on either side of the threshold is described. It led to the cure of the living person and the soul of the dead person.

27. An interesting study on the topic of support groups for cancer patients was published in the *New England Journal of Medicine* on 13.12.2001. The same issue also contains an editorial on the subject. The study and the editorial that responds to it sum up a dispute that has raged for some twenty years regarding the importance and extent of the influence of support groups on the treatment of people with cancer. What makes the results of the study particularly convincing is the fact that the researchers actually hoped to prove that support groups do affect the life expectancy of the sick person. As we said, the psychological results of the support groups suffice to justify their existence, even if their effect on the disease itself is less common. In contrast, diseases that are located in the soul body or life body can, in certain cases, be positively influenced by social support (Note #19).

28. The spiritual foundations of the curative education movement are found in the lecture series: *Education for Special Needs*, Rudolf Steiner Press.

29. More people have had spiritual experiences in the last decades not because spiritual experiences have become easier to attain, but rather because the karma of those people prepared them for it by means of the tests they underwent in their present or past lives. The aim of Anthroposophy, which entered overt human history a century ago, is to prepare humanity for the renewed encounter with the spiritual world, which began during the twentieth century and will increase in the future.

30. Structured exercises that are used as a preparation for meditation appear in the chapter: "Knowledge of Higher Worlds – Initiation", in the book: *An Outline of Esoteric Science*, SteinerBooks. They are also described in a slightly different way in the chapter, "Some Effects of Initiation", in the book: *How to Know Higher Worlds*, SteinerBooks. In the same book, the first chapter features a description, unequalled in its clarity and beauty, of the general soul qualities that are needed by the person who aspires to the spirit.

31. There are several "short cuts" by means of which a person can have spiritual experiences without going through all the stages of the preparation. Hallucinogenic drugs are an example of a short cut that exposes the person to danger to his mental health. Methods that employ physical asceticism are also liable to lead to serious consequences in young and sensitive people.